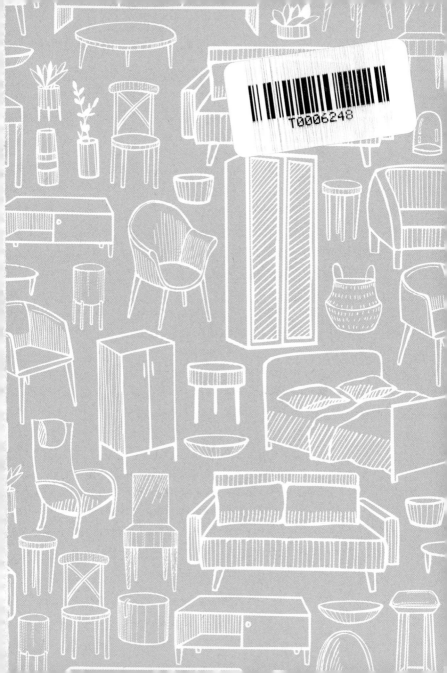

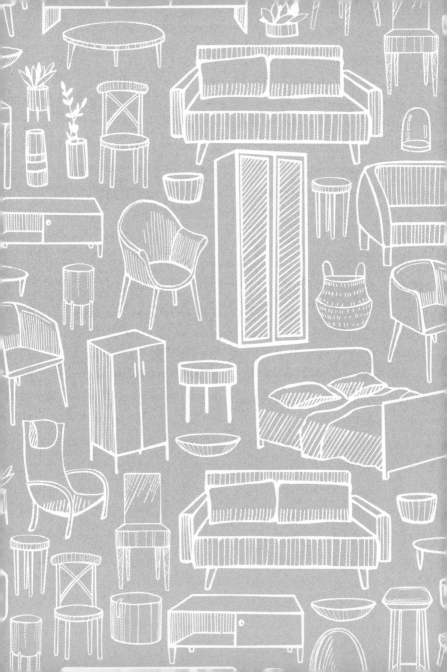

Praise for *Change Your Space to Change Your Life*

"Julie is truly a special, unique, and talented designer who has devoted her career to learning from the most valued master teachers about the art of placement, known as Feng Shui. Her ability to understand these ancient teachings is of great benefit to her clients during these modern-day challenges. Combining her knowledge of design, Feng Shui flow ideas, and a pure heart, her book reveals these qualities that can be incorporated into your living and working spaces." —**Caroline Patrick Bor-Nei, master educator of Feng Shui and author of** *Diary of a Feng Shui Consultant and Visual Artist*

"Julie Ann Segal's fun and practical approach to Feng Shui will inspire you to create spaces that raise your vibration and support positive growth in your life. Her approach to the art of Feng Shui makes the design process simple, lovable, and easy to follow." —**Mike Dooley,** *New York Times* **bestselling author of** *Infinite Possibilities*

"In *Change Your Space to Change Your Life*, Julie gives a very practical approach in mixing known ancient tools together with a crisp designer's wisdom and instructs how you can enhance your life by altering your personal environment and, in turn, creating the greatest life you ever dreamed possible." —**James Van Praagh, master teacher and spiritual medium**

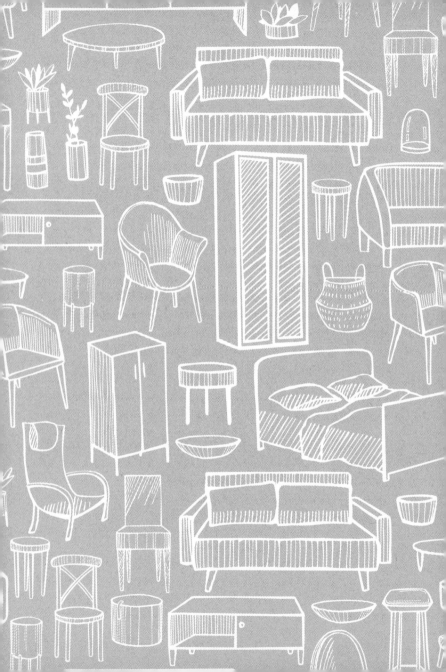

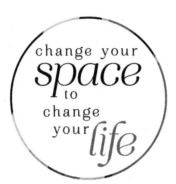

change your *space* to change your *life*

About the Author

Julie Ann Segal is an interior designer, Feng Shui consultant, and the owner and president of the design firm Metro Interiors. She received her BFA in Interior Design from Northern Illinois University and has served on the advisory board for the Century College Interior Design Program. She is certified as a Feng Shui consultant through the Wind and Water School of Feng Shui and is a member of the International Feng Shui Guild and the Feng Shui Institute of the Midwest. Learn more at MetroInteriors.com.

Julie Ann enjoys spending time with her four grown children and their families. She keeps active by practicing yoga, meditating, and running in nature. In her spare time, she loves to travel, try new recipes, and oil paint.

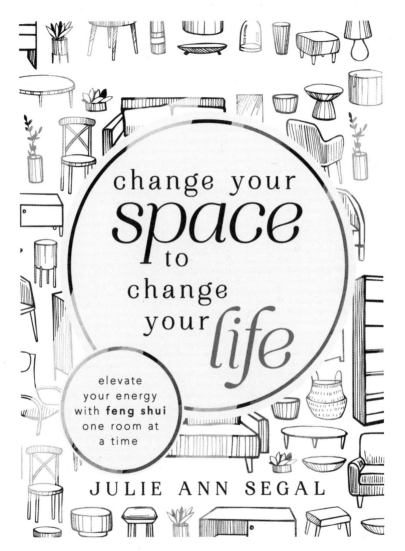

change your
space
to
change
your *life*

elevate
your energy
with **feng shui**
one room at
a time

JULIE ANN SEGAL

Llewellyn Publications | Woodbury, Minnesota

FIRST EDITION
First Printing, 2023

Book design by Christine Ha
Cover design by Cassie Willett
Interior art by the Llewellyn Art Department

Llewellyn Publications is a registered trademark of Llewellyn Worldwide Ltd.

Library of Congress Cataloging-in-Publication Data (Pending)
Library of Congress Cataloging-in-Publication Data

Names: Segal, Julie Ann, 1964- author.
Title: Change your space to change your life : elevate your energy with
   feng shui one room at a time / by Julie Ann Segal.
Description: First edition. | Woodbury, MN : Llewellyn Publications, [2023]
   | Includes bibliographical references. | Summary: "This approachable
   guide to Feng Shui-centered interior design sits at the intersection of
   spirituality, energy work, aesthetics, and personal connection. It not
   only provides room-by-room guidance, but also focuses on the big
   picture-the interplay between goals, intentions, and mindful design
   choices"-- Provided by publisher.
Identifiers: LCCN 2023011630 | ISBN 9780738774770 (paperback) | ISBN
   9780738775579 (ebook)
Subjects: LCSH: Feng shui. | Feng shui in interior decoration.
Classification: LCC BF1779.F4 S38 2023 | DDC 133.3/337--dc23/eng/20230503
LC record available at https://lccn.loc.gov/2023011630

Llewellyn Worldwide Ltd. does not participate in, endorse, or have any authority or responsibility concerning private business transactions between our authors and the public.
   All mail addressed to the author is forwarded but the publisher cannot, unless specifically instructed by the author, give out an address or phone number.
   Any internet references contained in this work are current at publication time, but the publisher cannot guarantee that a specific location will continue to be maintained. Please refer to the publisher's website for links to authors' websites and other sources.

Llewellyn Publications
A Division of Llewellyn Worldwide Ltd.
2143 Wooddale Drive
Woodbury, MN 55125-2989
www.llewellyn.com

Printed in the United States of America

Disclaimer

This book is not intended to prescribe, diagnose, treat, or cure any condition, and readers are advised to seek local and professional medical care for conditions that may be unique. Always be mindful when following generally stated medical advice; a reader's personal history, habits, and condition may alter results.

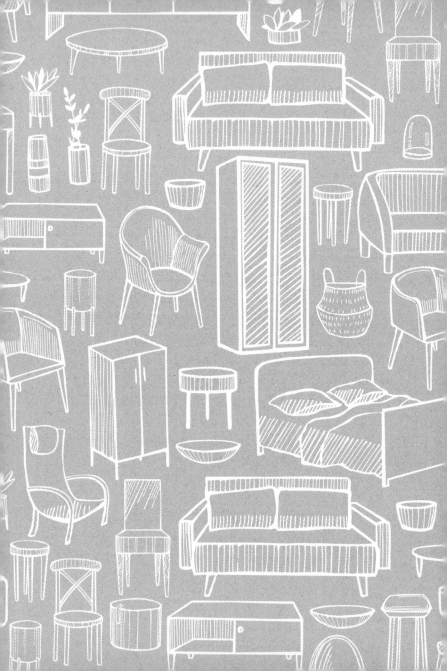

Acknowledgments

"The only impossible journey is the one you never begin."
—Tony Robbins

My journey started with the thought that someday I would write a book. At the time, I was a teenager. It took much learning and patience, numerous experiences, and many wonderful, uplifting, and supportive people to make that dream a reality.

To my mom, who is always there for me. Thank you for the days you spent writing with me and helping me express myself accurately. Your love and support always shine through, and I will forever be grateful for your selfless acts of kindness.

To Carole Hyder, my Feng Shui teacher. I am so thankful that you brought Feng Shui teachings to the Midwest. Your wisdom and knowledge inspired me to become the person I am today.

Thank you to Jessica Hoelzel, Jessica Staszak Abitz, Deirdre Van Nest, and Laura Zats, who helped organize my thoughts and narrate my ideas and stories. I appreciate your guidance and how much you taught me.

A special thanks to my personal editor, Kate Leibfried, for her countless hours of work to help me express myself. Your knowledge and talent contributed so much to this book. Your kind and nurturing demeanor helped me more than you know.

Thank you, Wendy Adamson, Nancy Meyer, and Ellen Sue Stern for your much-needed advice and encouragement.

My gratitude to all my clients for trusting me to design your spaces. I'm thankful for your permission to use some of your stories in this book. Thank you for believing in me and allowing me to live my passion. You taught me a great deal as I worked with each one of you.

I want to thank all my friends and family who have encouraged me to go forward and have given me the confidence to follow my truest path.

Thank you to my publisher, Llewellyn Worldwide, for acknowledging the significance of this content and for publishing my book.

Contents

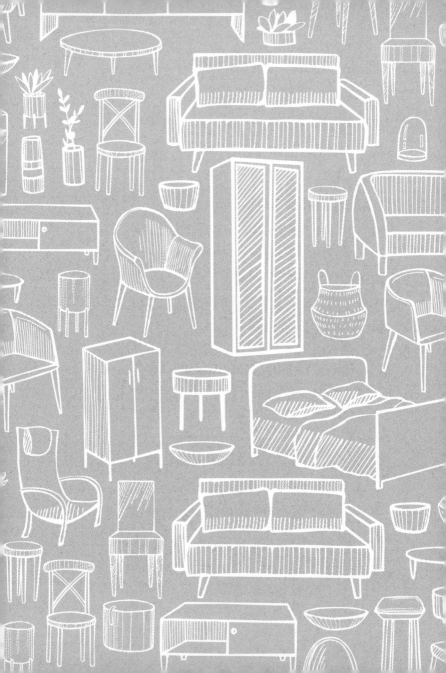

Foreword

In 1992 when I first heard about Feng Shui, it was a new concept to this part of the world. Although it has a four thousand-plus-year history, it didn't come to the United States until 1986 when a Buddhist lama introduced the idea that your space can reflect the condition of your life.

His Holiness Grandmaster Thomas Lin Yun moved from Taiwan to California to teach Americans about Buddhism, Feng Shui being part of the curriculum. Early on he assessed the differences between Eastern ideology and American perspective. As a result, he married the traditional concept of Chinese Feng Shui with psychology, architecture, interior design, and Western culture, making Feng Shui what it is today.

All of us who studied with him were encouraged to spread the word about Feng Shui and what it could do, adapting it as needed and adjusting the tradition when necessary but keeping the overall intention of helping people to live better.

This philosophy of adaptation influenced the twenty-three years of training I provided to more than five hundred students. Obviously the Western lifestyle didn't always fit the parameters of original Feng Shui concepts. He encouraged us to apply what we could from a traditional perspective and add what was needed from a more modern approach. His ideas were radical and came under fire from the purists, but he persevered, as did those of us who had the honor of studying with him.

In line with his encouragement to adjust and adapt within the traditional parameters, Julie Ann has taken the principles of Feng Shui and beautifully applied them to her field of excellence: interior design. She has written a respectful and informative book on how to put Feng Shui principles into a space that also subscribes to good design principles. Whereas many interior designers have quietly applied these principles in a client's space, Julie Ann has fearlessly stepped forward—Feng Shui has become a significant part of her message.

There's a Chinese saying that states, "Something is so purple that it's red." It means that something has acquired so much insight and presence that it changes into something better. The other way to say that is, "The student has surpassed the teacher." Indeed, Julie Ann has taken her years of study with me and others and has made it into something more.

Every interior designer should, of course, read *Change Your Space to Change Your Life*, but she has written it so anyone can benefit enormously from her approach. She weaves in the principles of biophilic design, the power of intention, the five Chinese elements, green design, sustainability, and inner knowledge and how all these fit into the paradigm of Feng

Shui. I am enormously proud of her accomplishments in the design field and in her latest effort to educate people about the power of Feng Shui.

Carole Hyder
Feng Shui master, speaker, teacher, author
Founder of the Feng Shui Institute of the Midwest

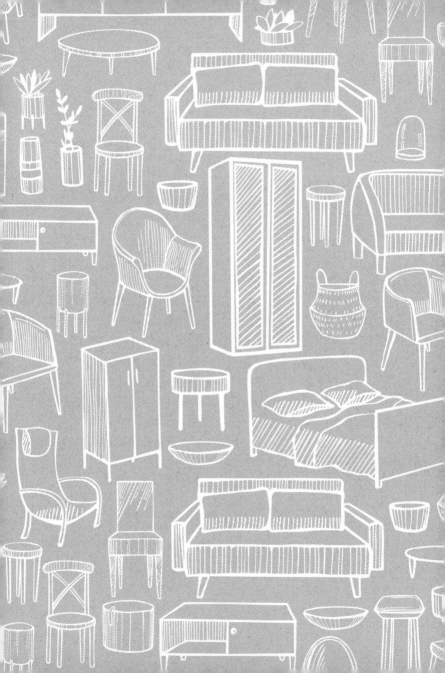

Introduction

My inspiration and excitement for life come from an inner knowing that there is more to living than what we can physically see and touch. We can tap into that knowledge not only through intuition and the mystical arts but by becoming more aware of the seeming coincidences of everyday life. Whether we realize it or not, we regularly encounter signs and symbols that can guide us toward happiness and fulfillment. When we are mindful of our thoughts and environment, we can make the appropriate changes to live our dreams and find fulfillment. When viewed this way, our surroundings become a fun and exciting playground.

My Story

As a young child, I would sit in my bedroom and try to figure out what would make it feel good—feel *right*. I intuitively understood that if my bedroom felt good, I would also feel good. With almost no budget for decorating, I spent time decluttering, rearranging my room, and adding blacklight posters until my bedroom resonated with me. Blacklight posters were popular in the 1970s and fit within my limited budget. I have come a long way with my resource library since then!

Starting college, I enrolled in the School of Business. At that time, I was inspired to build my own business, yet business courses did not resonate with me. Something felt off, but I couldn't quite put my finger on the cause of my disquiet. Then, something happened that changed my direction.

After winter break of my freshman year, I discovered my roommate's parents had transferred her to a different school. I had enjoyed my first roommate, and the news left me feeling disappointed and anxious. As an experienced sophomore, she had helped me navigate college life and inspired me to be a kind and respectful person. I felt safe and protected with her by my side.

When I walked into my dorm room that cold January day after winter break, I noticed I had a new roommate. She had decorated her side of the room beautifully. I saw a pretty floral bedspread with framed prints to coordinate and lovely accessories. I had not met her yet but was intrigued by her decorating skills.

My mom, who had driven me back to campus, knew how much I liked my former roommate and empathized with my situation. To cheer me up, she decided we would decorate my side of the room. So, off to JCPenney we went. We had fun browsing the department store and selecting new bedding, poster prints, and plants.

The next day at breakfast, my mom suggested that I consider interior design as a career path. "It is more than decorating," she explained. "It involves space planning, creating lighting plans, color palettes, and much more." She reminded me of how I spent my childhood rearranging my room and drawing pictures of rooms with furniture. The next day, I decided to look into shifting my courses to begin studying interior design.

I discovered the Interior Design Department was in the School of Fine Arts. In high school, my art teachers and mentors encouraged me to continue with my art, yet I wasn't confident I could make a living in that field. Now, I finally saw a path forward—a practical way to combine my love of art with a career. Once I switched my major to interior design, I began taking classes that involved drawing, painting, and color. I felt much more comfortable in these classes than in my accounting and finance courses. College finally became fun and exciting for me.

After graduating with a Bachelor of Arts degree with an emphasis in interior design, I gained experience by working in interior design companies before eventually opening my own business, Metro Interiors, in Minneapolis, Minnesota, in 1992. Though I enjoyed my work, I felt as though something were missing—some piece that would elevate my business to the next level. That missing element came to me in 2001 when I listened to a local presentation on Feng Shui (pronounced FUNG SHWAY) at an American Society of Interior Designers (ASID) meeting.

Carole Hyder and Barbara Bobrowitz copresented on the basic principles of Feng Shui and how those principles intertwined with interior design. I was enthralled. The presentation sparked my interest, and something about Feng Shui felt familiar to me. I had, after all, learned to trust my intuition as a young girl—to rearrange my furniture or place things around my room that made sense to me instinctively. Feng Shui seemed like the embodiment of some of my natural inclinations. I also felt drawn to Feng Shui Master Carole Hyder and knew she would become an important part of my life's path.

One of my friends had listened to the same presentation at the ASID meeting, and she felt equally compelled by Feng Shui. So, together we dove in! We learned what we could from books and articles and began spreading our limited knowledge in small informational sessions. I soon realized, however, that I needed to expand my knowledge of the multilayered world of Feng Shui. I decided to enroll in Carole Hyder's proprietary Feng Shui program to earn my certification.

Carole became a valuable instructor and mentor during the two-year program while I gained insight and developed essential skills to integrate Feng Shui into my business. She remains a teacher, colleague, and friend to this day.

Soon after gaining my Feng Shui certification, I joined the Feng Shui Institute of the Midwest and also earned certification as a Red Ribbon Professional of the International Feng Shui Guild (a distinction only given to those who pass the Guild's rigorous test).

Armed with a strong educational background in Feng Shui, I began to incorporate the skills I had learned into my interior design practice. It felt natural and intuitive. I began paying attention to subtle aspects of design and trusting my natural talents. The lessons I had learned during my Feng Shui courses made me a better designer who was more in tune with each space *and* my clients' needs. It wasn't long before my business began to receive recognition and became more prosperous than ever.

What Is Feng Shui?

At this point, you may be wondering what defines Feng Shui. To put it simply, Feng Shui is a four thousand-year-old Chinese philosophy used to create balance and harmony within ourselves and our environments through the art of placement. *Feng* means "wind" and *Shui* means "water," which are two important elements in this practice (we'll discuss the elements in detail in chapter 4). There are two main branches of Feng Shui: classical and modern. The classical version (sometimes called "compass") typically involves complex calculations relating to compass directions, occupants' birthdates, and more. These calculations are also used to identify specific energy areas of the home, known as the Bagua. The modern version, which is what I practice, is more flexible and does not use compass directions to guide design decisions. When mapping a home's energy, I also use the Bagua (discussed in chapter 8) but align the chart with the home's entryway. The version of Feng Shui I practice was popularized by Professor Thomas Lin Yun of Taiwan and is known as Black Hat or Black Sect Tantric Buddhist Feng Shui (sometimes called BTB).

The root of Feng Shui involves creating harmony within our interior spaces *and* between our interior spaces and ourselves. Our health, well-being, happiness, and prosperity are integrally tied to our surroundings. Picture walking into a workplace with buzzing white lights, blank walls, no windows, and uncomfortable seating. How does such an environment make you feel? Anxious, perhaps, or full of melancholy? Such a space is certainly not nurturing or inspiring.

The instinctual feelings you get from your surroundings are directly tied to the essence of Feng Shui. Your environment can influence you, whether you realize it or not. A poorly planned space will probably have draining, detrimental side effects, whereas an intentionally planned space can motivate and uplift you. Feng Shui can assist in creating the enriching, nurturing environments we all crave.

Who Can Practice Feng Shui?

Sometimes my clients are intimidated by Feng Shui. They feel overwhelmed by its many layers and protocols. In truth, there's nothing to fear. Incorporating Feng Shui into your space can be lighthearted and exciting. That's why I call my approach the "Fun Shui Way." I combine this art of placement with full-service interior design and make it fun and approachable for my clients.

My intention in writing this book is to make Feng Shui enjoyable and accessible to people of all backgrounds and experiences. Even those with no prior design knowledge can use this book as a guide to adjust or redesign an existing space—or create an entirely new one. This is not a glossary of Feng Shui terms or an encyclopedia of Feng Shui practices. Even though I provide useful tips and best practices to overhaul or adjust your space, I will *not* cover every single aspect of Feng Shui (this book would have to be at least a thousand pages to do so!). I believe it is much more important for you to learn essential Feng Shui principles that can be applied to many different circumstances and spaces than to learn, for instance, the specific principles of smoky quartz. That said, I will dive into plenty of examples and stories throughout this book to illustrate the principles I am teaching and help bring the narrative to life.

What We'll Cover in This Book

Our journey begins with a discussion about energy—that everpresent force that surrounds and guides us. The energy of a room is tangible and can have a direct effect on our mental and emotional well-being. We then move into a chapter on goal setting (one of the foundational components of any effective design) before discussing the various tools required to successfully utilize Feng Shui in design (hint: *you* and your intentions are two of the most important tools).

After covering these foundations, we will begin to explore Feng Shui essentials, including creating a balanced space, properly utilizing the five elements, space clearing and decluttering, and tapping into the power of colors and symbols to create a comfortable home or workspace that reflects *you* and your intentions. We will also discuss ways to incorporate powerful natural elements into any room through the practice of biophilic design. The section on Feng Shui essentials concludes with an introduction to the Bagua—a system that divides a space into nine energetically distinct areas and guides us to adjust and improve each section. This potent tool may seem intimidating for those unfamiliar with it, but I intentionally wrote this chapter to be user-friendly and filled it with practical examples.

The book concludes with chapters that focus on creating healthy changes and adjusting your space to fit your ever-changing life. Human beings are not stagnant—we flow and change like a river—and it's important to have our living spaces reflect who we are and who we would like to become.

Where are you in your personal journey? What dreams and aspirations do you have for yourself? Feng Shui–focused design can help you manifest and achieve your personal goals and improve the energy of your home or office, which, in turn, can improve your well-being and plant the seeds for positive change.

Though Feng Shui can facilitate amazing transformations, it is *not* the same as calling upon a genie in a bottle. Rather, it is an ancient, intentional practice that taps into the natural energy of a space and channels its flow in a productive, positive way. Though it takes years to become a trained Feng Shui consultant, anyone can master the basics with a little studying, a willingness to make intentional improvements, and an open heart. Let's begin (and don't forget to have fun!).

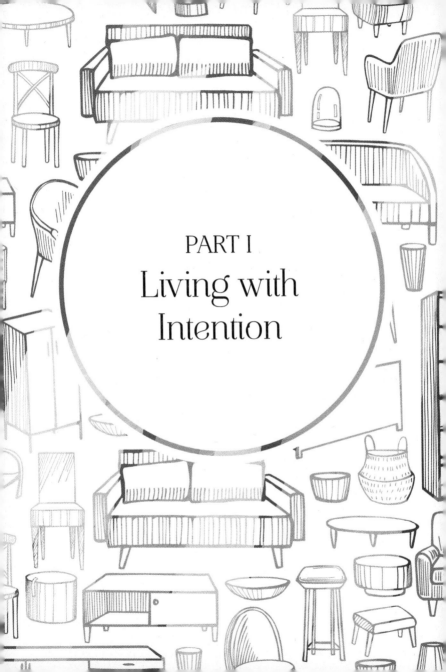

PART I
Living with
Intention

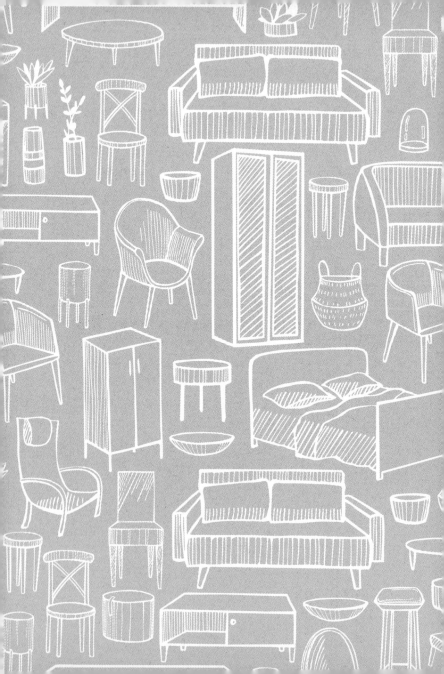

Chapter 1
What Is Energy?

There is a common misunderstanding that material objects are inherently unspiritual. However, our material possessions can carry profound importance to us, and we can tap into their energy, or chi, through mindfulness. This chapter will provide a primer on how energy flows through space and the way it affects our lives. Energy exists in and between everything in the world. Anything you can touch—your coffee table, your dog, the lemon on your counter, your foot—is composed of atoms. Atoms are constantly in motion with electrons whirring around neutrons and protons. This constant motion—this *energy*—is everywhere on Earth, including in our homes. And it is energy that can make us feel either connected to or disconnected from any given space.

The philosophy of Feng Shui emphasizes that everything is energy and everything is connected. Quantum physics has shown us that our entire world and, indeed, the known universe is composed of energy. We are surrounded by an energy field that experiences constant motion and vibrations. Feng Shui consultants have understood energy (chi) intuitively for thousands of years, and the study of quantum physics is beginning to prove what Feng Shui consultants have long known: we are all part of a great universal energy field and are intimately connected to each other and to our surroundings.

The International Feng Shui Guild's Glossary of Universal Feng Shui Terms uses energy as a blanket term to refer to all forms of chi, or a universal life force that exists everywhere.[1] It is the movement of life force within our living space or body that can affect our well-being either auspiciously or inauspiciously.

Energy in Spaces

The way a room makes us feel (its energy) can have an impact on how we show up in the world. When we go out to a business meeting or a social event, the room itself can have an uplifting or sobering effect. We have the power to create environments that bring comfort and enhance our lives. It matters not the size of your living or working space, whether you have an abundance of expensive possessions or live modestly. Positive energy can be found in whatever makes you feel healthy, happy, and alive.

Imagine you spend a good portion of your time in a drab, undecorated apartment filled with clutter and lacking sunlight. The walls are stark white with nicks. The furniture is stained and broken, and the carpet is worn out. What do you

---

1. Ashdown, Prinzivalli, and Jampolsky, *The International Feng Shui Guild's Glossary of Universal Feng Shui Terms*, 22.

feel when you think about this type of room? Are you feeling depressed, confused, uncomfortable, distracted, or out of balance? Those feelings are natural in a space such as this.

Now imagine a room that is beautiful to you. When I do this, I see a living room that is open and full of life. The room has large windows with colorful draped fabric panels and blinds to control the sunlight. The space is bedecked with a balanced arrangement of comfortable furniture and fun wooden storage pieces, which store only items I use and love. Beneath my feet is a soft, textured carpet; on the walls are a few pieces of artwork that make me smile. Green, healthy plants and a few accessories adorn the room. Now what are you feeling? Do you feel joyful, peaceful, or energized? Are you experiencing physical and mental clarity?

Spending a lot of time in the first room would undoubtedly affect your energy. It would drag you down and may even bring out your worst features. However, the second room I described would likely have a positive effect. It would help you feel energized, peaceful, and happy. Energy tends to follow you out of your space and into your relationships. It impacts how you react in life, whether with your kids, coworkers, or the grocery clerk.

As a Feng Shui consultant, clients often ask me what it means, exactly, to have "good energy" in a home and how to create it. The way I define energy, in simple terms, is how your space feels. If you have clutter, broken or worn pieces, and haven't paid attention to the design or your furniture arrangement, the space may not feel right to you. Even if you own beautiful things—attractive furniture or sophisticated paintings, for instance—it *still* may not resonate with you. Something might feel "off." Trust your intuition when it comes to perceiving energy.

In reality, energy is neither good nor bad. It's what we associate with the way we feel. Most of us want to feel uplifted and supported. These feelings help us move through life more positively and improve our daily experiences and interactions. Living in homes and working in offices where we set up our space with intention enables us to feel comfortable, positive, energized, and motivated. Therefore, we can change our lives by changing our space. This illustrates the basic Feng Shui principle that our space reflects our lives.

An out-of-balance bedroom, home office, or family room could create an imbalance within ourselves, even if we are not aware of what is causing this feeling. A peaceful space can enhance our feelings of serenity. When we take the time to work on inner harmony, it's a good idea to create a space that reflects this energy. Otherwise, our hard-earned gains may be difficult to maintain, and our sense of well-being may slowly erode.

I once visited a friend who lived out of state. When I walked into her apartment, I saw she had no art decorating her rooms, and the walls were painted stark white. She said she could never decide on paint colors or artwork, so she never bothered to hang anything or paint the walls. She also confessed that she was continually moving her furniture around but was never satisfied with how it looked. I sensed (and this was later confirmed) that she was having difficulty with her self-worth and was lacking clarity in her life. Her inner world was suffering, and she had not been paying attention to her personal well-being.

As I walked into the living room, I noticed her metal blinds were old and worn, and many were bent at odd angles. Looking at them, I felt as though they were old bandages clinging to the home's interior, and they gave me the impression that the apartment was sick or suffering.

Intuitively I felt that the home's condition could have a negative impact on my friend. I pushed the thought aside, but it came rushing back a few minutes later when she told me she had been grappling with a skin disease. There is little doubt in my mind that the apartment's state (lacking color and neglected) had amplified this illness.

Like my friend, many of us underestimate the impact of our surroundings on our bodies and minds. If we take the time to create an environment that pleases us, it will uplift our spirits and contribute to improved health and well-being. Our health and relationships are negatively affected when we ignore our surroundings, and we may begin to feel tired and depleted. Another factor that contributes to a lack of well-being is clutter.

Energy and Clutter

We can experience clutter in many different ways. Clutter occurs when too many items are packed into a small space or when things are disorganized or untidy. Clutter can be defined as an accumulation of things you rarely use or no longer love. It can also consist of anything unfinished—that half-crocheted quilt in the closet, for example, or the letter you never mailed to your ex. Clutter can also be mental, emotional, or spiritual (how many times have you felt overwhelmed by negative thoughts or emotions?).

No matter how you define it, clutter has a significant impact on the Feng Shui of your space. It can hold you back in the past, block opportunities, and clog the natural flow of energy. Most importantly, it can affect your health—physically, mentally, emotionally, and spiritually. Everything you own takes up space in your mind and body, whether you realize it or not. The clutter in your house or apartment isn't just a metaphor; it has a real-life impact on your mental clarity, personal energy, and well-being. It doesn't matter if the clutter is tucked away in a closet. Your subconscious *knows* the clutter is there.

Think about something as simple as the junk drawer. When it's packed to the brim with a mishmash of random items, that brings your energy down. You might have to dig through piles of rubber bands and twist ties, packing tape, and craft supplies just to find whatever it is you need. This not only wastes time but can lead to frustration and anger. It makes you want to give up the search as soon as you begin.

Now imagine the drawer has been cleaned and reorganized. You tossed all the items you didn't need, put away objects that belonged elsewhere, and only kept the supplies you use frequently. Now when you open the drawer, you can easily see what you have and find everything with ease. When I do this in my own home, I feel my energy flow more freely, and I move more positively throughout my day.

How would this feel if you could extend this type of order throughout your living space—entryway, kitchen, laundry room, bedroom, home office? How would that affect your life overall?

One clutter-cutting technique you can try is filling one paper grocery bag each week with items you no longer use or love. Place each filled bag in your garage or storage room for a period of time—perhaps a month or two. If you discover you did not need or miss those items during that time, that signals it is time to release them. Use this method for as long as you need, until you have significantly cut down on household clutter.

One of my clients, Harriet, was recently divorced when we met. Although she was heartbroken and depressed, she would not openly express those feelings. We worked together to create rooms that were aesthetically appealing and dramatic, using the finest materials and furnishings available. After we completed the spaces, giving attention to every detail, Harriet would go online and order boxes of unnecessary items she impulsively liked at the moment. Many boxes remained unopened, and soon her home began to fill with clutter, which gradually took over the newly designed spaces. As her large home became closed in with "stuff," her body started developing circulatory problems. As the energy in her home became constricted, her body started to constrict as well, further demonstrating how our inner being and outer surroundings reflect each other. She also became withdrawn from the outside world, which negatively affected her relationships. Harriet's residence began to mirror her inner state of depression and loss. She was trying to fill the space outside of herself with material things, but it was never enough. With counseling, Harriet was able to make the connection that material things cannot compensate for working on your feelings, thoughts, and beliefs.

As seen in Harriet's case, clutter overwhelms us and holds us back from realizing positive change in our lives. Clutter can make us feel bogged down, anxious, or drained of energy. On the other hand, when an individual works on improving mentally, physically, and emotionally, they can more easily create a lighter, more pleasing environment, which reflects this healthier attitude.

Self-awareness and self-improvement work in tandem with Feng Shui. As you begin to improve your space, you can gain more energy and clarity to improve your life, and vice versa. In this way, Feng Shui is very much a holistic practice. It takes into account the personal aspirations of the occupant as well as best practices for creating balance, harmony, and energy flow in a space.

Your Turn

Following are three recommendations to create harmonious energy. When we pay attention to these fundamentals, we start to cultivate the chi, or energy, in our space, creating a more comfortable area for living and working.

1. **Allow for flow/movement in your space and prevent stagnant or blocking energy.**
   Take a walk through your home. Do certain rooms feel crowded with furniture, knickknacks, or other items? Are objects placed behind doors or obstructing natural walkways, thereby blocking energy? Does your furniture arrangement appear inviting, or are certain pieces preventing you from moving freely in the room?

2. **Surround yourself with what you love so it resonates with your vibration (doesn't feel "off").**
   Think about your home. Does it reflect meaningful memories from the past? Does it also reflect the person you are today *and* who you want

to become? Are you holding on to objects you haven't used in years, that hold no meaning for you, or that have negative associations? Letting go of items that are unused, broken, or no longer speak to you can free up time, energy, and space.

3. **Motivate and energize yourself.**
   Use this renewed energy to propel your self-improvement journey. Remember: Your mind and body are intrinsically linked to your space. Treat your body as you would your home— with love and respect. That means tuning in to its needs, nourishing it, and understanding when you need to make changes.

   For me, one of the self-improvement changes I made was to significantly reduce my gluten intake. I am sensitive to gluten, and when I eat it, I become bloated and anxious, which makes it difficult to sleep. I feel more relaxed and sleep better when I do not eat foods containing gluten. My increased energy has made all the difference in the world when it comes to the performance of my daily activities. The spaces where we live and work affect our body and energy levels, just like the foods we choose to eat.

Paying attention to these fundamentals can be an excellent start in cultivating the chi/energy in your space so it not only looks good but feels good too. When your space gives you a sense of contentment, it is working to support you in your life.

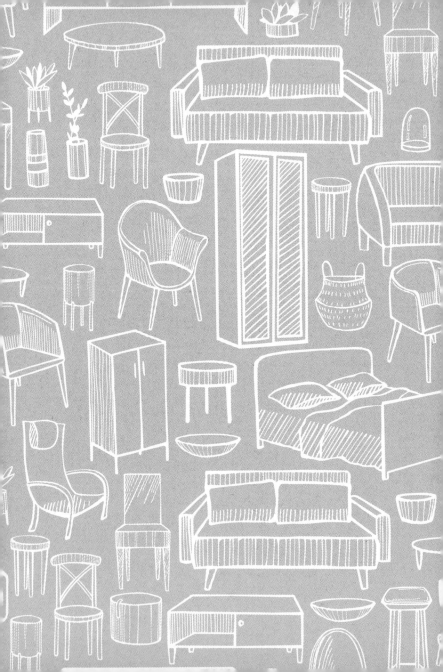

Chapter 2
Designing with Goals

W hat would you like to change in your life? We all want more or less of something. More money, less stress. More romance, less conflict. More career advancement, less illness. When you bring a Feng Shui perspective into your design, you can align your space with what you truly desire. Adjusting the Feng Shui can make an incredible difference.

Before we can effect change through design, we must clarify our desires and set well-defined goals and intentions. After clarifying your goals, you can begin to make Feng Shui adjustments, which can be incorporated into the planning stages of the design. When you make thoughtful decisions and plan accordingly, positive energy is set into motion and supports you, whether you are consciously thinking about it or not. Keep in mind, Feng Shui is not a one-size-fits-all practice. The adjustments you make to a space should be personalized to match your current circumstances and goals.

Using Goals to Direct Design

The following story is about my client, John, and his daughter Sarah and how they reached their goals by making changes in their home after John's divorce. Before I began designing, I talked to John about what he wanted in his own life and what was important to him.

John, a successful businessman in his late forties and newly divorced, contacted me for a home design consultation. Sarah had medium-length brown hair and a pleasant smile. She was cordial but had a bit of an attitude toward her dad, as many teenagers do.

Like most parents, John was concerned with Sarah's happiness and well-being but also worried about her growing distant. He said, "I'm afraid she won't want to spend any time here in my home." His main goal, therefore, was to create a welcoming, comfortable environment that would encourage Sarah to spend quality time in their house and foster a positive father-daughter relationship.

John made it clear to me that he didn't have a flair for design and confessed he was scared about starting the process. He said, "What if I do all this, spend the money, and it doesn't work out? What if Sarah doesn't like it?"

I was the second designer John had hired, and he was hesitant about the outcome. Fortunately, John's desire to have a great relationship with his daughter outweighed his fears. We decided to move forward with one room—the basement.

"I want this to be Sarah's special place," John said. He wanted to create an area where she could be comfortable, have friends over, and feel relaxed. Ultimately he hoped she would want to spend more time in the house with him. Sarah was on board and excited by the prospect of having her own place for sleepovers, hanging out with friends, and playing games. And she wanted purple walls!

At that time, the basement was musty smelling with worn, stained carpeting and furniture. The walls were stark white with contrasting, dark woodwork and small windows that added little natural light. The energy felt stagnant and draining—not an atmosphere that encouraged people to spend time there. Because of this, the space was neglected and scarcely used.

When it came to transforming the space, Sarah was involved with design choices every step of the way. In most cases at Metro Interiors, we create a scaled floor plan on the computer so clients can see different furniture arrangements and space configurations. If the furniture fits on the floor plan, you can be confident it will fit into the room. It's much easier to move the furnishings around that way. Using these planning tools, along with my expertise and Sarah's natural talent for design, we began to transform the room.

To create the change and meet Sarah's requests, we chose a muted purple for the wall paint, balancing it out with creamy white beadboard wainscoting, which is vertically grooved paneling that runs partway up the wall. We installed larger windows, which brightened the room and allowed sunshine to illuminate the space. On the walls, we hung customized digital artwork that Sarah enjoyed. A pool table, comfy sofa, and a convenient built-in snack and beverage center created the perfect entertaining and hangout space for Sarah.

Four months after the project was completed, John called me and exclaimed, "I'm so happy! Sarah is using the room exactly as I'd pictured." She was hanging out with friends and spending more time in his home. His goal for transforming the room was realized, as was his desire to stay connected with his daughter. His worries about the process had dissipated. Sarah loved it, too, telling me, "It's amazing! It turned out so much better than I could have imagined."

I know we're talking about remodeling a room on the surface, but the more significant remodel was actually to their relationship. The furniture arrangement had a flow. No longer closed in or restrictive, it mirrored the change in John and Sarah's relationship, which became more open and harmonious.

Correcting an Underutilized Space

After the successful basement remodel, we started on the upstairs family room. This space was underutilized, and John's goal was to make it an inviting area for entertaining and family time. He had already spent several thousand dollars on an oversized, uncomfortable sofa and love seat. "They are too deep, and the room feels cold," John complained. "Because of that, nobody likes to sit here long. And no one wants to eat here either because the fabric is white!"

The room was experiencing additional problems as well. The light blue rug was soft but added no interest to the room. The TV equipment did not look aesthetically pleasing in its cabinet, and the TV hung awkwardly in the corner. John was frustrated and wondered if I could make it better since he could not envision a solution.

To start, we decluttered the top of the mantel and added artwork that popped along with a few statement accessory pieces. We chose a soft custom wool rug with colors that coordinated with the room and added interest. We ordered a comfortable leather sectional to provide more seating and practicality. The sofa was open for easy TV viewing and small enough that we could place an additional chair in the room. To conceal the unsightly TV equipment, I custom designed a corner cabinet to contain it. We left the TV in its original spot, but with the corner cabinet directly underneath it, it became more visually clean and grounded.

With the Fun Shui Way, everything in your space becomes a metaphor for your life. For example, making a TV feel more grounded by adding a cabinet underneath it can help *you* feel more grounded. Making noticeable changes in your space can change your life.

Resisting Change

Throughout this project, John would become concerned since he had already spent money on household furnishings and designs that hadn't worked out. Now he was trying again and wondering if it would make a difference. It is natural for people to be hesitant when they're making significant changes that will affect their lives. Has that ever happened to you? Have you ever known something was the right decision for you but pulled back because of fear?

In the middle of redesigning John's family room, I didn't hear from him for three months. When John finally answered my call, I could tell he was ready for change. He had just needed time to process things and move forward. So we continued with the project, making sure Sarah signed off on any proposed changes. Once we finally completed the room, John was thrilled with the results. He blurted out, "I can't believe it! Now, Sarah's spending time here with me, watching sports on TV, having snacks, and entertaining friends." The changes made the room more usable, visually cleaner, nicer looking, and more grounded. It also became more comfortable and conducive for entertaining. John told me how pleased he was with the transformation and thanked me for being so patient. He said it was an excellent process for all of us. We transformed the space using the *Fun* Shui Way.

Think about your own home or office. Are there underutilized areas or spaces that are not living up to their potential? Do they feel "low energy" or "off"? Could the spaces be improved in terms of functionality or aesthetics? These observations can point to ways you could make changes to benefit your life. Identifying potential problem areas is the first step toward consciously changing your space to change your life—improving it for yourself and those you love.

Sometimes it's as simple as adding a bench where you never had one before to make life flow a little easier for you. Changing little things that often get ignored can make a big difference in your happiness. Another example is adding a mirror to expand your space. With the right intention, this action can also be a metaphor for expanding or growing something in your life. What do you want to grow and develop? Chapter 8 teaches the Bagua basics, which is a tool that can be overlaid on a blueprint to learn how areas on the map correspond with areas of your life. For example, you can find the "career area" of your home and place a mirror in that room to grow your career. Making changes with intention can have a profound impact on your life.

Conscious Design Changes

A year later, I got another call from John. This time, he said their dining room was not working. They were not comfortable eating there, and papers and books tended to pile up on the table. "I don't know what's wrong," he said, "but you know how to help me, and I want you to do your *Fun* Shui thing." By this point, John had no hesitation and completely trusted the process.

So, we set a goal to create a more comfortable, welcoming space that would be used regularly. At the time, the dining room *appeared* to work functionally with a rectangular table and six dining chairs. To add life to this space, I had already added a floral arrangement and a new light fixture in addition to hanging a piece of artwork John already owned. But something was still off; the space felt closed-in and unwelcoming. It was time to improve the dining room's functionality and aesthetics, just as we had done with the previous rooms.

My solution for John's dining room was to use a round table to open up the room. Using a round table also creates a feeling of relaxation, whereas a rectangular table can feel confrontational. With a round table, you're sitting *around* the table together rather than sitting face-to-face. Circular shapes add softness and help bring balance to a room. We also added a warm window treatment, a silk birch tree, and colorful contemporary art.

I knew we accomplished our mission when I stopped by one day to drop something off and noticed the new table was free of papers and books but did have a few crumbs on it. John told me he was not only pleased with the redesigned dining room, but he and Sarah were throwing dinner parties together and using the room as intended.

Think about your own life and your own living space for a moment. Are there any changes you can make to build stronger relationships with your family members like John and Sarah did? John had initially furnished and decorated his place on his own and noticed it wasn't working or that parts were "just okay." How is your space? Is it working, or does it feel "just okay"? Does the energy feel off? Use your observations to set goals for yourself and your space.

John's story relates back to the main message of this book: if you want to change your life, it's helpful to make conscious changes to your space. If you plan carefully and intentionally, as John did, you can positively influence your life's path.

Start with Decluttering

If one of your goals is to improve your energy level and happiness, a great way to foster those positive changes is to start decluttering. You can redecorate all you want, but it won't make much of a difference if your home is jam-packed with stuff. I mentioned decluttering in chapter 1, but it bears repeating: eliminating clutter is *key* when it comes to fostering positive energy and creating a nurturing, uplifting environment.

This is especially true if you live in a smaller space, such as a studio or one-bedroom apartment. In this case, you'll have to be especially mindful of which items to keep (useful items or things that give you joy) and which to rehome or discard. If an apartment is overly cluttered, the energy will not flow properly, and you will likely not want to spend much time in your space.

In the case of single-family homes, it makes me sad that so many people only declutter and fix up their homes to sell them when they could fix their homes to enjoy for themselves. Besides, if you're constantly improving and adjusting your home, you won't have to fix it quickly when you *are* ready to sell. This can be a major stress reducer in the long run.

As you declutter and set about making changes in your space, keep your goals and desires at the front of your mind. Before beginning a redesign, it is essential to clarify what you want—your overarching objectives. You *can* create a better world and, more precisely, envision the way you want to be in this world. There are no right or wrong answers. *Your* answer is accurate.

Your Turn

To open your mind to your deepest desires and awaken your awareness of possibilities for your life, try implementing the following meditative writing exercise. This exercise will help clarify your goals and guide you in your design changes.

To prepare, set aside a block of time or small blocks of time that are free from distractions. Consider doing this exercise a little at a time so you don't feel pressured.

Sit quietly for about five minutes and relax. Focus on your breathing and let go of any pressure. You can handle whatever thoughts surface later. This experience is intended to be a fun and expansive activity.

Once you're in a relaxed state, begin to write. In no particular order, answer the following questions:

1. **Who or what do you want to *be*?**

   Think about how you feel each day, your purpose or mission, how you show up in life, your
   strongest traits, the kind of parent/partner/
   leader you are, etc. If you love certain traits about
   yourself, include those as well. Write "I am"
   statements and add details.

   EXAMPLE: I am thoughtful. I am confident.
   I am a brave leader. I am wealthy. I am compas-
   sionate. I share my generous spirit with others.
   I am a positive role model. I am a sought-after
   interior designer. I am a world-class speaker.

2. **What do you want to *do*?**

   Do you want to travel, start a business, or offer a
   new program in your current business? Do you
   hope to spend more time in nature, get married, have kids, play, or learn a new skill? Write
   out your desires in descriptive sentences or as a
   list. Write as if you are *already doing these things*.
   Explore the options. Don't limit yourself in
   any way.

   EXAMPLE: I travel to Paris and spend
   two weeks exploring the city. My classes are
   immensely popular and make a huge positive
   impact in my clients' lives. I create exciting and

fun spaces for people to live and work in. I speak French fluently.

3. **What do you want to *have*?**

Perhaps you would like a vacation home, more free time, a new car, or several new outfits. Let yourself dream big. Many people get a little freaked out and feel greedy if they admit to wanting. It doesn't feel "noble." Open yourself to those "have" desires. Knowing what they are can guide you to the places where you resist, block, or sabotage your success.

EXAMPLE: I have all the time in the world to travel. I have a spouse who adores me. My funds are working for me in my retirement investments. I have money to support the growth of my business. I have clients all over the world whose lives are benefiting from our work together.

Chapter 3
Intentions and Tools
for Improving Results

Practicing Feng Shui is not only about selecting the right color of wallpaper or the right texture and shape for a chair. It's not only about placing a bookshelf here or a table there to harmonize the energy of the room or to increase happiness and prosperity. A key factor in making Feng Shui work to your advantage is making sure your life force, or chi, is aligned with these physical changes.

The most fundamental lesson of Feng Shui is that our physical spaces have profound effects on our mental states, and vice versa. A broken doorknob can set off arguments between family members or make us testy with friends or even strangers. But we can't fix what we don't know is broken. If we want to usher positive changes into our lives, we need to understand how to harness awareness and positive thinking to achieve it.

Just as our environments can affect our health and well-being, so, too, can our mental and emotional health influence the decisions we make for our spaces. An uncluttered, peaceful mind is more likely to make sound choices regarding re-arranging or adjusting a room (or an entire home or office).

By putting your mind in the right space for change, you will become better able to set intentions.

Intention Setting in Feng Shui

The difference between goal setting and intention setting is subtle but important. Goals have more to do with results and future projections. They are often specific and easy to visualize. Intentions, on the other hand, have to do with the energy you are projecting and your frame of mind. Your intentions may be specific, but oftentimes they are broader or more nebulous than goals. For example, you might *intend* to live a healthier life and thus set *goals* to eat a healthier diet, meditate, or move your body every day.

In yogic practices, an intention is known as a *Sankalpa*, a term that combines two words, *san*, meaning "a connection with the highest truth," and *kalpa*, meaning "vow."[2] Therefore, an intention can be thought of as a vow to achieve one's highest truth. Intentions are a compass; goals are the end points.

Intention setting and Feng Shui are intrinsically linked. If your intentions are not clear or sincere, it will be difficult to effectively change your space. It is important to maintain positive thoughts to keep your energy elevated and your intentions pure. If you feel down or drained of power, not only will you not feel driven to accomplish your goals, but you won't attract the energy you need to help you accomplish them either.

---

2. McGonigal, "How to Create a Sankalpa," *Yoga International*.

When you feel called upon to make a change—whether that change involves finding a partner, spending more time with your family, or blazing a path into a new career—Feng Shui can help you turn those aspirations into a physical reality. Using the appropriate tools to uplift your energy will help you get into the right mental attitude to create your desired outcome.

Keep in mind, your actions matter, too. Be an active participant in your destiny and use intention setting to propel you forward. Sometimes that may involve asking for what you want. Just as you might call upon the universe for assistance and guidance, it is sometimes necessary to call upon other people for their advice or aid. The universe is ready to help, but you need to do your part as well!

When I was a kid, I imagined having my own business. This dream began when my mom's friend gave me a personality test that told me I would make a good entrepreneur. I did not know what owning a business involved or what kind of company I wanted, but I latched onto the idea and started telling people I would someday run my own business. I repeated that idea so many times over the years, it became a strong internal belief. Friends and family heard my words and started affirming that I would have my own business. With this belief guiding my path, I started my own design firm only a few years after graduating from college. My experience isn't the only proof I've had that thoughts (coupled with action) can change the world. Many clients and colleagues have come to the same conclusion: whatever you repetitively think about with intensity can become your reality.

The problem is, both positive and negative thoughts can manifest into reality if given enough attention. When I started my business in 1992, I used to play a game. Whenever I reached a monthly sales goal, I would reward myself with a piece of jewelry, a new outfit, or even a piece of furniture for my home. This game motivated me to reach my goals by using a fun approach instead of focusing on the stress of running a business. However, when a friend of mine found out about this game, she laughed at me. She thought it was ridiculous to reward myself for work. I felt ashamed and embarrassed, and for a while, I quit playing the game.

Not long after that conversation, my sales started to decline. Looking back, I realized my friend was struggling in her own life. Her lack of belief in herself meant she didn't feel good enough to reward herself with such gifts. Lack of professional fulfillment and monetary success were external stressors that were creating negativity within her personal space, and she was projecting that negativity onto me.

When I realized I had also taken on harmful beliefs, I began taking steps to regain my freedom and empowerment. I understood how vital those rewards had been in building my self-confidence, and I began to play the game again, which returned success to my business.

Understanding your patterns of thought and how words can become a reality is essential to understanding what physical changes need to take place. Consistent thoughts become concrete manifestations, and when they are in alignment with your intentions, you have a match made in heaven. Changing your thought patterns takes time, practice, and patience. You must be willing to look closely at the beliefs you hold about yourself and the world and the limits those beliefs can set on your actions.

Five Energy Tools

This chapter contains five energy tools for self-reflection, improving mindset, and setting intentions: vision boards, journaling, breathing exercises, words of affirmation, and wind chimes. These tools are designed to help you examine your thought patterns; understand how those thought patterns affect your actions, intentions, and goals; and begin to turn them into more positive and supportive beliefs.

If you want to clarify your intentions, try journaling or making a vision board. If you'd like to feel more centered, relaxed, and energized, try using the breathing technique. And if you want to strengthen your connection to the universe and your subconscious mind, try using wind chimes or writing a list of affirmations (like the ones provided at the end of this chapter). In addition, I recommend adding a breathing or meditation practice to your daily routine to center yourself regularly.

The clearer your intentions, the easier it will be to see your space with fresh eyes and perceive its potential. When you keep your intentions in mind, you should gain an understanding of a room's possibilities and how it could change to better serve the person you are and the person you want to be. For example, if your intentions mainly center on improving family relationships, keep that in mind when modifying a room. Are the chairs arranged to easily facilitate conversation? Are the color choices, lighting, and artwork bright and cheerful? Is clutter kept at a minimum so people will actually *want* to be in the room? All of these insights can be gained by keeping your main intention (in this case, family relationships) at the forefront of your mind.

Before you can apply Feng Shui principles to your life, you not only have to know what you want, as we discussed in chapter 2, but you must also mentally prepare to make these changes. Refer back to this chapter when you want to choose a tool to help you get into the proper mindset to set your intentions.

Vision Boards

What is a vision board? A vision board is a surface on which you display images that represent circumstances or events that you want to happen. It is one of many tools for visualizing your intentions and getting you into the right frame of mind to achieve them. It can include drawings, photographs, or words that describe the things you would like to acquire or accomplish, such as buying a home or going on a nice vacation with your partner. You may find and clip images from magazines, the internet, or promotional ads. For my vision board, I sometimes use a decorative bulletin board on which I pin the images that match my goals and desires. If you can't find a beautiful-looking, ready-made bulletin board, most frame shops can make one out of corkboard and a decorative frame of your choosing. Using poster board or foam core and glue works well, too. I once glued my images right onto a painter's palette. It is also possible to make a digital vision board, although I would make sure to post it in a spot you view every day, such as the background of your computer screen.

Over the years, many of my clients and friends have had a lot of fun setting their intentions (and exercising their creativity!) while making vision boards, and they have had amazing results, producing cars, vacations, and promotions as well as increased joy, happiness, and love. In terms of Feng Shui, visualization or vision boards can help you achieve your home or office improvement goals. How do you want your space to *feel?* If you're hoping to remodel or redecorate your kitchen, for example, try browsing through pictures of kitchens and adding the ones that evoke joy or inspire you. Perhaps you're entranced by a certain color palette or the way a room is laid out. Don't overthink it. Trust your instincts and add feel-good spaces to your board.

I teach vision board classes and have seen my students succeed with this process. Maya, one of my students, added wooden carvings to her vision board. Not long after, she started a new venture making homemade wood art carvings. Her mind was creating based on what she had put on her vision board, even after she had forgotten she had selected that image. The vision board helped her turn her dream into reality.

Take a look at the Be-Do-Have statements you wrote at the end of chapter 2. Search for images that represent your statements. For example, if you wrote about finding more peace in your life, look for a picture of a peace sign or a tranquil landscape to use on your vision board—whatever evokes "peace" to you.

When I am getting dressed in the morning, I spend a few minutes looking at my vision board, internalizing the images and imagining how I will feel when my dreams come true. I also let go of how my dreams will happen. Often, we get what we want in unexpected ways, and visualizing specifics can limit your view. One philosophy I've picked up and embraced is that the cursed "hows" will get in the way. Instead of focusing on *how* you will accomplish your goals, surrender the details and let the universe lead you. I've used this technique many times, including during my Infinite Impossibilities Certification Training in Santa Fe, New Mexico.

The Infinite Impossibilities program, developed by spiritual leader Mike Dooley, is designed to teach us how to create an ideal life by examining our thoughts, beliefs, emotions, and intuition. To complete my training, I went to a conference in 2017 with many other trainers from every walk of life, all sharing a spiritual drive to live with an awareness of their thoughts, beliefs, emotions, and intuition and to make intentional changes. As Infinite Impossibilities trainers, we guide others through this deliberate approach to life.

When we arrived, the leaders of the conference announced a contest for the most inspiring and fun social media posting. During the meeting, I got so wrapped up in my training, I forgot about the competition. Even so, I enjoyed posting and interacting online and did so almost subconsciously. I hadn't planned to win the contest, but I did anyway!

After I returned home from the conference, I noticed I had placed images on my vision board about six months earlier of a woman taking photos with her smartphone (a symbol I had chosen for improving my social media presence). I had also selected a picture of a star with the words "Only One Star" written on it (a symbol I had chosen for becoming a social media star). I would imagine posting compelling photographs with the right words to convey my experiences creatively. By seeing these images daily and internalizing the intention to improve my social media presence, I was subconsciously put in a mindset that helped lead to my success in the Santa Fe contest.

With visualization, it is essential to get into a positive, upbeat emotional state—the way you will feel when you receive the desired result. When you place an item on your vision board, try to imagine that your goal has already come true. Acting as if the outcome already happened is one way to achieve your desired goals. You'll likely find that you'll be bolder, more confident, and feel more resolute if you decide to proceed as if success is inevitable.

In addition to visualizing outcomes, I have found that awareness, openness, and gratitude are all key aspects of intention setting. When I am consciously aware of the synchronicities happening in my life, my heart opens, and I become grateful to the energy of the universe. Genuine gratitude helps keep you feeling positive, motivated, and joyful. Use these techniques and this frame of mind when you're creating your vision board to change both your life and your space.

Journaling

Journaling is another powerful tool for getting into the right mental attitude to set your intentions and thus achieve your goals. As someone with a lot of project ideas and the drive to accomplish them all, I am very aware of how crucial it is to obtain focus. Without focus, it is nearly impossible to bring major intentions and goals to fruition. You'll likely find yourself spinning in circles, frustrated, and not achieving much forward motion. By writing down your thoughts and aspirations in a journal, you can examine and assess them to find which ones are the most important to you and thus discover where you should place your focus. You may wish to set aside a special notebook for your journal entries or create a particular folder on your laptop. You could even utilize a special software program to organize your journaling, such as Penzu, Scrivener, or MacJournal.

When you journal, try not to focus on the writing itself. Do not edit as you go or worry about proper grammar or punctuation. The point is to let ideas flow from your pen or keyboard, not to get hung up on your usage of semicolons! When you write, let your thoughts flow. You might set aside a certain amount of time every day to journal. Even ten or fifteen minutes is enough time to establish a healthy writing practice.

After my divorce, I found myself trying to accomplish too many things at once while also maintaining a dating life. I was out of balance and having a difficult time focusing and remaining centered. On the advice of my life coach, Michelle, I began to reflect on what was important to me and what I wanted in my life. I decided to write about the type of man I sought to be my future partner. I wrote about how I would feel comfortable, secure, and at peace with him. He would be generous with his time, helpful around the house, and affectionate and passionate with me.

But I didn't know how to make this vision a reality until Michelle asked me how I could become an ideal partner. I probably wouldn't find what I was seeking until I worked on myself first. Being as honest as possible, I started writing about how I would become a better partner. By writing about the actions I would take for my future partner, I gained perspective on my role in a relationship. Men are human, too, I thought, and one can't expect everything to come from them! I began to understand my blind spots, and I realized I needed to work on listening to my partner's needs and think about what more I could offer in a relationship. I also reflected on my strengths, which included supporting my partner's dreams and ambitions, communication, and unconditional love.

I had a couple of long-term relationships shortly after my divorce and then went through a myriad of dates; some became friends, some were casual, others were painful. What I was learning throughout this period was the delicate balance between being realistic and being discerning. Out of the confusion and commotion, I became a stronger person and realized I am whole and do not need a partner, but I choose and like the idea of sharing life with another person. While setting unrealistic expectations can lead to an unhealthy relationship, the right relationship can help each partner grow while sharing the joys and pressures of life between them.

Eight years after my divorce, I asked my life coach, Michelle, to help me gain clarity once again. Upon reviewing my past journal entries envisioning my perfect partner, I realized a lot of the men I had dated did not match many of the qualities I had written down. Michelle asked me to make a list of all the qualities I had described in my journal. When I finished, I separated the characteristics into two columns: "must have" and "nice to have."

As I unearthed these insights through journaling, I also began to make changes in my living space. Keeping my intentions top of mind, I began creating space and reorganizing my bedroom to make room for another individual. I cleared out closet space so another set of clothing could hang there. I made sure there was a nightstand on both sides of the bed with a lamp on each one. I purchased artwork that evoked a harmonious couple—for example, a painting of a chair next to a hammock, which represents a place for two people.

Within a month, I met someone who met my criteria, and we both fell in love. This relationship lasted three years, and even though it ended, the journaling, reflection, and space clearing helped me find clarity. He had many of the qualities I had written about—much more than those in my previous relationships. Journaling helped reveal insights that allowed me to make meaningful changes in my space and thus make room for a successful relationship.

Breathing Techniques to Increase Chi (Life Force)

Breathing techniques are an excellent tool to help you get unstuck in your life and create the energy, flow, and clarity you need to accomplish your goals and intentions. There are times in all our lives when we feel vulnerable and out of control. For me, one of those times occurred after my divorce in 2009. At first, my confidence was running high: business was great, friends were plentiful, and I had the freedom to travel to fun and exotic places. But in 2013 I suffered a personal crash. I had a string of bad relationships that year, and at the end of each one, I spiraled further downward, feeling more and more out of control. This crash culminated with my dad's passing. After losing my dad, I began to shut down and started to feel numb.

At that point, I called upon Patrick, a yoga and meditation teacher with whom I had worked in recent years. The most powerful practice I learned from Patrick was his technique called Unlimited Breath. Before we started, he would give me half an hour to vent my frustrations, my fears, my hopes, and my desires. Then we would begin the process of letting them go.

Patrick had me lie down on a massage table and get comfortable, directing my attention to my breathing. We did not communicate much, except when Patrick needed to direct my breathing, encouraging me to breathe deeper or slow my pace, and I focused solely on my breathing. When we finished the hour-long practice, I felt an immense release of frustration, pain, and exhaustion from my body. During that hour, those emotions were replaced with a sense of joy, acceptance, and peace. I felt relaxed and energized at the same time and ready to live in the moment. It is quite honestly the best high in the world (and without any harmful side effects).

The effects of this breathing technique are caused by taking in plenty of oxygen. Some people worry that taking in too much oxygen will cause hyperventilation, but hyperventilation happens when we exhale more than we inhale, which depletes carbon dioxide levels and can cause a number of harmful symptoms. Shallow breathing increases tension, anxiety, and panic attacks. Breathing deeply and exhaling slowly, on the other hand, slows the heart rate and calms the nerves.

Breathing habits can have an enormous impact on health and well-being.[3] Breathing not only provides us with energy but releases toxins through our exhalations. Becoming consciously aware of your breathing habits can both significantly decrease stress and provide moments of peace during which you can focus and find clarity. When practicing this technique, it is difficult to concentrate on your breath and think at the same time. Increasing your oxygen intake and freeing your mind by focusing on breathing allows the subconscious mind to take over, which can reveal old wounds and trauma and release any blockages in energy.

The clarity gained from this type of profound breathing can lead to important breakthroughs about who you are, who you want to be, and what changes you need to make to get there. And when your intentions are clear, it is easier to effectively practice Feng Shui. After all, Feng Shui is largely about intentions and making mindful modifications to your space

---

3. André, "Proper Breathing Brings Better Health," *Scientific American*.

to improve your life. Self-improvement and understanding are vital components of the journey. You must work to improve and adjust your inner world, just as you might work to improve your outer world—the spaces and environments that contain us each and every day.

When getting started with the Unlimited Breath technique, it is essential for a practitioner to walk you through the breathing methods and keep you focused. Your breath is a powerful force, and the way you breathe can have profound effects on your emotional and mental state. Because of this profound power, it is vital to perform the technique correctly.

Start by lying flat on your back and getting comfortable. You can use a pillow under your knees or a blanket over your body to situate yourself in a restful position. Begin by breathing from your upper chest only, taking in deep breaths and releasing them through your mouth at a quick but steady pace so you hear the sound of the breath going in and out of your body. Continue this breathing process for approximately forty-five minutes to an hour (beginners may choose to start with a shorter session—whatever is comfortable for you).

If you start feeling light-headed and tingly during these sessions, don't worry. These are normal sensations. During one of my first experiences with this breathing technique, I became so tired I thought I could not go on. Patrick responded by pointing out that this is how I felt about my life—that it was too hard and I was too tired. He encouraged me to continue to breathe through it. That was a big eye-opener. I hadn't been aware of my feelings that life was too hard and tiring, but I had somehow expressed those subconscious thoughts through my breathing. This process enabled me to identify those harmful thoughts and change them—to begin thinking of life as easy and start seeing myself as awake and alive.

While performing this technique, you may also experience a popping sensation in your body or heaviness in certain areas, but don't worry. These sensations are often followed by an incredible feeling of lightness and freedom.

For me, this release helped heal the trauma I felt in 2013 from lost relationships and the passing of my father. By becoming more in tune with my breath, I became more balanced within myself. I began an internal healing process in which I could let go of past wrongs and realign my expectations. As a result, I was able to bring this newfound clarity into my interior design and Feng Shui work. I was in a better mental and emotional state to create pleasant, peaceful designs centered around intention.

Affirmations

I moved my interior design business to a small Victorian home in Minneapolis, Minnesota, when my marriage was beginning to fail, and I desperately needed a space to improve my focus and grow my business. The house was on a hill, and behind it was another hill—an auspicious and protective location for a building, according to Feng Shui practice. During the last year I rented the office, I ended up living there as we sold our family home. The downstairs became my workspace; the upstairs, my living quarters. With an uncertain financial future, I ended up living alone, without my kids, for six months. While I felt sad and lonely in the small house, it gave me time to grieve my old life while also allowing me to dream of the future. In the evenings, I would go upstairs to my cozy living space and write affirmations about my new life.

Affirmations are positive and uplifting statements meant to manifest a better life or pave the way to a better future. Consistently saying or writing affirming statements about your ideal future can help lead to the desired result. Acting as if the statements have already come true strengthens the process. Constant repetition of affirmations retrains your conscious and subconscious mind to think differently and accept the statements as though they are already a reality. It takes practice and patience to do this, but when you feel as though your statements are already a reality, your energy changes and begins to work toward your intentions. The clearer you are about what you want (which is vital when practicing Feng Shui), the more likely it will happen.

To write affirmations, start by jotting down some changes you want to make in your life. Turn those changes into positive and uplifting statements in the present tense. If you need help getting started, go back to the Be-Do-Have exercise from chapter 2. For example, if you would like to find a romantic partner but are having a difficult time believing it can happen, you could write an affirmation like this: "I now have a happy and fulfilling romantic relationship." If you are shy and think it is hard to make friends, you could write an affirmation like this: "I easily talk to people and effortlessly make friends at parties and social events." Taking the time to write affirmations will clarify your path and give you the fortification you need to make necessary changes in your life *and* your space.

The following are examples of some of my favorite affirmations:

1. I trust the process of life; all is well in my world.

2. I choose foods that are nutritious and healthy for me.

3. I am prosperous; money flows freely to me.

Louise Hay, author of bestselling books such as *You Can Heal Your Life* and *Meditations to Heal Your Life*, was a pioneer in working with affirmations to heal physical ailments and mental disorders. She spread awareness of the mind-body connection through her writings and her practice. Louise's books are powerful and wide reaching and have been translated into multiple languages. Reading *You Can Heal Your Life* as a teenager started me on the path toward creating my best life. When things got tough, I often turned to her lessons.

Graduating from college and venturing into the real world, I was fearful about many things. When I began my interior design career, I constantly wondered if I was good enough to succeed. Would I get any clients? Would people like my designs? Was I creative enough? My list of fears went on and on.

A few affirmations I wrote in my twenties helped give me strength and confidence at the beginning of my career and, ultimately, became my reality. I wrote the following statements and repeated them often:

- I easily and effortlessly guide my clients through the process; I work with them to overcome blocks or barriers.
- I am positive and enthusiastic when working with clients.
- My career is working perfectly.

Another time I used affirmations to achieve success was in my late thirties. At the time, I had just given birth to my fourth and youngest child. I love my kids dearly, but it was not easy with four small children, a career, and a divorce lurking in the shadows. I longed to feel freedom, happiness, joy, and adventure again—feelings I embodied while on vacation.

During this time, I was enjoying the art of beading and began creating a line of beaded bookmarks and keychains I called "Every Day's a Vacation Bookmarks and Keychains." This name was an affirmation I would read over and over as I created and made tags for these items. With every repetition of that affirmation, I brought the thought of "everyday vacations" into my consciousness. These daily mantras manifested into an incredible opportunity.

A client, Jane, hired me to work on her home in the Minneapolis area. Then she decided to buy a second home in southern California along the coastal highway in Laguna Beach. It was right in the middle of what one might call "Vacationland." After she bought her vacation home, she began sending me there three or four times a year to help create a balanced and Feng Shui–centric design. One day, I realized that even though I was remodeling someone else's home, I was having a blast! Plus, I was right on the beach. My time in Laguna Beach never felt like work; it felt as if every day was a vacation. I had achieved the goals I had defined in my affirmations.

You can create your own affirmations, find inspiration online, or read motivational books to help spark ideas for affirmations. Repeat your affirmations a few times each day, either by writing them in your journal or speaking them out loud. As you repeat them, visualize the statement and imagine it is already true. Soon, you will feel as if it *is* already true. If you don't give up and do continue to imagine yourself in the world of your affirmations, you will one day find yourself living that truth.

Wind Chimes and Bells

In 2002 I moved into a new home with my three kids and husband. My husband did not usually play an active role in the household, so I found myself taking charge of all the packing and unpacking. I was in the middle of working through my Feng Shui certification class and was trying to put my training into action. However, it was difficult juggling childcare, unpacking, and studying at the same time, and my business was not getting the attention it needed. After several months of living in our new home, my business had become stagnant. My husband was not supportive of my endeavors, criticized my homemaking and childcare decisions, and bemoaned the unpacked boxes (despite his own unwillingness to help).

What I learned at the Wind & Water School of Feng Shui helped me through this difficult time: when you change your space, your life changes, too. I had not yet mastered the art of becoming fully aware and conscious of the inner life I could create with and through my physical home, and I was beginning to feel completely out of control. I knew it was time to start implementing my training in my own life, and I decided to start by getting my business unstuck.

My first step involved making a Feng Shui adjustment. I hung a metal wind chime above my desk chair where I would sit to do my interior design work. Metal is one of the five elements in Feng Shui and generates energy for focus and provides clarity. At the same time, it dissipates negative energy. Hanging it was a visual symbol, and it helped me change my thoughts and affirm focus and clarity. I knew it was working when I started to become more organized and began making business calls again. I would regularly reach up and ring the wind chimes while keeping an intention in mind, which would serve to strengthen that intention.

Wind chimes are also used in Feng Shui to call in or ask for what is needed from the universe. When I rang the chimes above my desk, I would ask for more clients. That was the main intention I put out into the universe. The very week I began using wind chimes, I received a call from a man who owned a property management company and was interested in my services. I had met him years prior and had wanted to work for him, but he had failed to return my calls or letters. Now, he was calling out of the blue and wanted to hire me to choose interior and exterior colors for his apartment buildings. Ultimately this new project led to him referring me to larger property management companies and to me designing multi-housing common areas, which became a substantial part of my business.

Through using the wind chime above my desk, I also received clarity about the placement of my office. I realized it was not set up in the right location—the energy felt off—and so I decided to relocate it to a room I had originally planned to use as my craft room. In this room, I could shut the door and have the privacy I required to concentrate and build my business. Having my office open to the family room had not been conducive to generating the right energy for work, as the family room is a place to entertain, watch TV, and relax. I added a fresh coat of paint, placed a custom-sized area rug to cover the hard vinyl tile floor, arranged my office furniture, and added some beautiful art to the room. My office began to take shape and feel comfortable. My focus sharpened and I was able to concentrate again.

Bells work in a similar way to chimes. Placing them in a proper Feng Shui location (as discussed in chapter 8) and ringing them with intention can call in what you need from the universe. When purchasing wind chimes, keep in mind that the tone, clarity, and sound are critical, and they should be pleasing to you. I keep a bell on the far left-hand corner of my desk, the area for wealth and abundance. Any time a check comes into my office, I ring the bell and place the check under it until I am ready to deposit it. You can do this, too. This energetic action keeps money flowing in, and it also helps me trust that I will have a prosperous future rather than being fearful of not having enough. Living in fear can push opportunities and wealth away from you.

Your Turn

The five energy tools I introduced in this chapter are far from the only tools you can use to lift yourself, get into a positive mindset, and gain clarity. Many other tools can be helpful, such as working with essential oils, candles, crystals, energy work, healing touch, tai chi, chi gong, and more. You can also utilize sensory tools associated with sound, light, water, and vibrations, which I will introduce in chapter 10.

In the meantime, try these three steps for achieving greater clarity and setting intentions:

1. **Practice listening to your intuition and acting upon your gut feelings.**
   While reflecting on your goals and ambitions, it is vital to listen to your inner knowledge and follow your hunches. I believe your gut feeling is always right, but thoughts and doubts sometimes get in the way, making it difficult to listen. Focusing on mental and physical health, in addition to clearing a path to a positive and uncluttered mind, will help you to sort out what—and, more importantly, *who*—is most important in your life. Once you achieve this clarity, you will have a better understanding of what you need to work toward with your Feng Shui adjustments. Keeping your intentions in mind allows you to experiment with purpose and target your creativity.

2. **Select at least one of the five energy tools described in this chapter and begin practicing it this week.**
   Consider which of the five actions—creating a vision board, journaling, using breathing techniques, writing affirmations, or using wind

chimes—will best serve you in the present moment and decide to work it into your routine.

3. **Develop a practice.**
   Whenever you're starting a new routine or discipline, consistency is key. Commit to your new energy work (one of the five actions listed in this chapter) by intentionally setting aside time each day to engage in your activity of choice. Block off your calendar, find a quiet place, and fully immerse yourself in your practice.

To create consciously and intentionally, we must continually make an effort to reflect on our inner lives and recenter ourselves. By using the tools I have laid out in this chapter, I hope you can find that balance for yourself. Remember: Your inner work is intrinsically linked to your external space. Keep this in mind as we begin to explore Feng Shui basics, starting with the five elements.

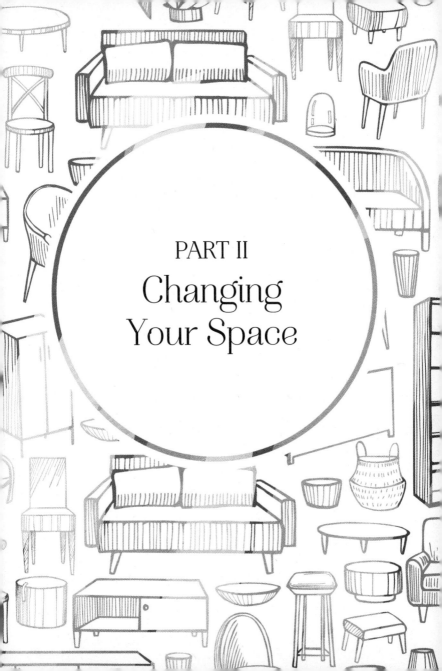

PART II
Changing Your Space

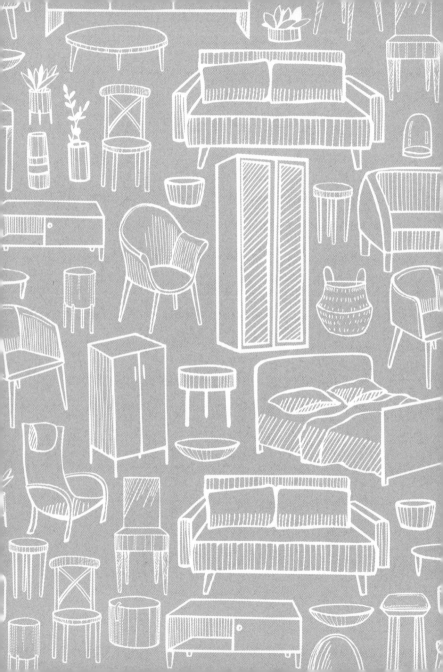

Chapter 4
Finding Balance

W hen embarking on the journey to change your space, it is important to begin with reflection. Think about each room in your home (or if you live in a modestly sized apartment, consider each distinct section of your space) and ask yourself these three essential questions:

- ✦ Does the room reflect who I am today?
- ✦ Does it reflect who I want to become?
- ✦ Am I living in the past?

The previous chapters emphasized taking time to find clarity and being deliberate about living with intention. These are the first steps in your Feng Shui journey. By gaining clarity on what's working and what's not, you can start the process of making positive changes to your physical space.

Creating Harmonious Spaces

When your space is in sync with who you are, this will usher in a sense of peace, joy, and balance. On the other hand, if your inner and outer worlds are not harmonious, your environment can cause you to feel unsettled or anxious. On top of that, an unbalanced environment can contribute to or build upon negative emotions. The home office of my client, Beth, is an example of how an unbalanced room can subconsciously stir up feelings of stress and disquiet.

I was first contacted by Beth and her husband, Steve, to help with their living room. But that changed during our first time working together. While showing me around, we looked at Beth's home office and discussed why it was not functioning well for her. When I viewed the space, I immediately noticed how heavy and cramped it felt. Too many large pieces of furniture and clutter overwhelmed the room and evoked feelings of claustrophobia.

I suggested that the office redesign take priority, especially when I discovered she worked from home full-time. The living room had a view of the cluttered office space, which created a feeling of discontent when trying to relax. I began to help Beth create a more productive working environment as well as a comfortable space where she could think more clearly and focus on her daily tasks. Additionally, by redesigning the office and removing the interference of a room in disarray, she and others could feel more relaxed in the living room.

The result was an impressive transformation. Beth reflected on the renovation, saying, "Before the redesign, my office was a disorganized mess that said nothing about me. I tended to use it as a catchall for things I didn't know what to do with. Now, it is well-organized, bright, and the layout seems to flow naturally."

To facilitate this change, Beth spent a lot of time decluttering, letting go of objects she didn't use or love. We also removed two large bookcases and a couch to clear the clutter and lighten the feel of the room. Oversized or undersized furniture or accessories can throw off the balance of your space—especially in a small room or an apartment—so it's important to consider the size of your pieces before placing them in a room.

After clearing the space, we chose a warm, soothing, neutral paint color for the walls, a cozy rug, and an upholstered chair, which created a relaxing reading area. A new painting with a bright and lively flower garden became a focal point. Beth delighted in the painting since gardening is one of her favorite hobbies.

We procured a desk that was less weighty but allowed for a larger workspace and also upgraded Beth's desk chair to a high-back leather one. The new desk was placed in the command position, a placement that is considered a position of power in Feng Shui. A table, bed, or desk may be placed in the command position, which is essentially when a particular piece of furniture is situated so it has a clear view of the door but is not directly aligned with it. This placement is about controlling your energy, not controlling others. For Beth, we intentionally placed her office desk in the command position to give her an enhanced feeling of control.

We also gave Beth plenty of storage. She now has easy access to the things she needs and uses frequently. For the windows, we replaced metal blinds with wooden roman shades for a more natural look and a lighter feel. We intentionally chose cordless blinds so nothing hangs in front of the beautiful backyard view.

The Five Elements

As we worked on Beth's home office, I made sure to keep the five elements in mind: fire, earth, metal, water, and wood. When these elements are in balance, a space will feel more harmonious and complete. In Beth's office, the elements were represented in various ways:

Fire was represented by a painting of a red and orange flower.

Earth appeared in the earth-toned accents we used and the color of the blinds.

Metal was represented by metal lamps and the use of the color white in artwork and chair fabric.

Water was conveyed through the wavy patterns of her artwork and through the water contained in a vase of fresh flowers on her desk.

Wood was represented by her wooden desk and plants.

In the end, we accomplished our goal of creating a space for Beth that was conducive to work and also enjoyable. She says, "My work attitude and feeling of what the office is has changed—I like to be there even when I'm not working. It doesn't *only* feel like an office but a relaxing place to be."

The five elements we incorporated into Beth's office are fundamental in Feng Shui. Each element embodies certain energies and has specific colors, shapes, and images associated with it. The following chart shows how each element can be represented and the impact they can make. When balanced within a room, the five elements can impact the people living or working there positively. When they are out of balance, they can negatively affect the occupants.

Feng Shui Elements
"The Five Elements"

WOOD

Shape: Columnar

Colors: Greens & blues

Energy:
- Expanding
- Growth
- Entrepreneurial

Object Examples:
- Real wood
- Plants
- Wicker
- Rattan

METAL

Shape: Circular

Colors: White & pastels

Energy:
- Detail-oriented
- Precision
- Refinement

Object Examples:
- All metals
- Dome shapes
- Metal sculptures

FIRE

Shape: Triangular

Color: Red

Energy:
- Active
- Passion
- Enthusiastic

Object Examples:
- Fireplaces
- Sunrise
- Stoves

WATER

Shapes: Wavy & irregular

Colors: Black & dark Blue

Energy:
- Meditative
- Reflective
- Inward

Object Examples:
- Mirrors
- Lakes, rivers, ponds & oceans
- Seashells

EARTH

Shape: Square

Colors: Yellow & earth tones

Energy:
- Stability
- Balance
- Grounding

Object Examples:
- Pottery & ceramics
- Food
- Rocks

TOO MUCH OF AN ELEMENT:

Fire: Agitative, explosive, mood swings & impulsive

Earth: Worry, over-protective & conservative

Metal: Rigid, fussy & obsessive with cleanliness

Water: Fearful, overwhelmed & spaciness

Wood: Hasty, driven & stubborn

TOO LITTLE OF AN ELEMENT:

Fire: Lack of originality, burned out & frigid

Earth: Selfish, insecure & feeling abandoned

Metal: Chronic anxiety, judgmental & fear of failure

Water: Narrow vision, unable to perform & anxiety

Wood: No strong opinions, nervous energy & easily frustrated

Have you ever seen a photo or been in a place mostly decorated in white? The room might have quality furnishings and look sophisticated, but it can feel cold and rigid. This is one of the effects of having too much metal energy present, as shown in the chart above. Now visualize adding plants, wooden furniture, a lovely shade of yellow on the walls, and a mixture of colors in the pillows and artwork to add warmth and to bring forth the other energies. These touches will balance out the overwhelming presence of metal energy in the space. On the other hand, if metal is lacking in a room, you may find yourself having difficulty focusing or concentrating. In this case, add a little more metal (through color choices, materials, objects, or shapes) to support your mental clarity.

Element Interactions

The five elements interact with each other in powerful ways. An element has the ability to either create or destroy other elements. Because of this, it is important to consider which elements are represented in your space and whether they are having a detrimental effect or a positive effect on another element.

For instance, water feeds wood (a positive effect). If you think about the relationship between water and trees, this makes logical sense. Other relationships are a little more abstract, such as the correlation between fire and earth. When fire burns to ash, it produces new earth. So, fire aids in the creation of earth. If you're in need of a little more earth/ grounding in your home, you could consider introducing fire instead. The option is yours, and it's best to do what feels intuitively correct.

You will, however, want to be mindful of the destructive effect elements can have on each other. Certain elements can counteract the effects you're trying to achieve when introduced to a space. For example, water extinguishes fire. If you're hoping to cultivate more fire energy in a particular area, it is best to avoid references to the water element. For more details on the relationship between the elements in terms of creation and destruction, please examine the following figures.

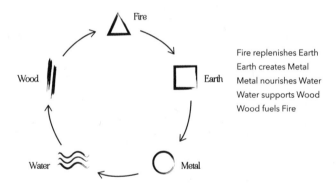

Fire replenishes Earth
Earth creates Metal
Metal nourishes Water
Water supports Wood
Wood fuels Fire

Figure 1: Creative Cycle

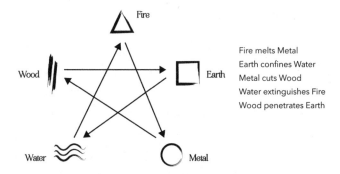

Fire melts Metal
Earth confines Water
Metal cuts Wood
Water extinguishes Fire
Wood penetrates Earth

Figure 2: Destructive Cycle

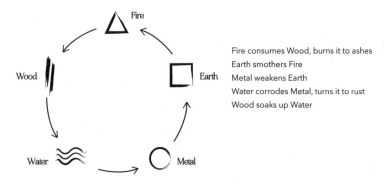

Fire consumes Wood, burns it to ashes
Earth smothers Fire
Metal weakens Earth
Water corrodes Metal, turns it to rust
Wood soaks up Water

Figure 3: Controlling Cycle

The five elements not only appear in our surroundings but also within ourselves. Each person embodies every element, though most of us embrace some elements more strongly than others. If you want to make changes in your home, it's a good idea to become in tune with yourself and begin to understand which elements are prominent in your personality. In addition to using the reflection and mindfulness methods discussed in chapters 2 and 3, consider taking a test to determine your dominant elements (these tests can be found online). In my case, I tend to have a lot of wood energy, which shows up in my entrepreneurship and my motivation to start new projects, and fire energy, which manifests in my passion, enthusiasm, and drive. Knowing this about myself, I make sure the other three elements are prominent in my space to balance out my natural wood and fire energy.

If you're unsure about your prevalent elements, that's okay. Above all, it is important to understand your weaknesses and strengths and to gain clarity around your goals and intentions. Pay attention and start to notice how you feel in a given room or an area of your home or office.

In 2018 I moved from a high-rise apartment on the six-teenth floor to a townhome on the ground. The change was dramatic. While living in the high-rise, I spent much of my time working and doing; I did not spend enough time *being*. I rarely cooked. I also went through a series of unhappy romantic relationships. It occurred to me after the move that

I did not have enough representations of the earth element in my space. I had plenty of wood, including green walls, wooden furniture, floors, and cabinets, and the wood element gave me the energy to start many projects and grow as a person. The fire, metal, and water elements were also present, but I was noticeably lacking earth.

I became distinctly aware of this deprivation when I moved to a new home on the ground. The difference was profound. I felt much more grounded, having the ability to walk directly outdoors and be in nature. I was especially delighted to see the leaves on the trees from my window. In my old space, I had to travel down sixteen floors to walk outside, and even though my view of the city was spectacular, I didn't realize I lacked the earth element until I moved.

For those who live several floors up in a high-rise building, you don't have to move to become more grounded. Instead, add earth objects or colors that represent the earth element to find balance. When I moved into my townhome, I added beautiful rocks and stones and even painted niches in my living room a deep golden yellow. I started to cook again and found relaxation by watching TV (something I had rarely done since my college years). Since I had more balance in my space, I felt happier and more grounded.

Yin and Yang Energy

Another Feng Shui balancing concept involves working with yin and yang energies in your space. Yin is feminine energy that embodies passivity and serenity. This type of energy can be found in internal stillness, the soft flow of water, or the dark silence of night. Yang is masculine energy that embodies action and movement. It can be found in the swift movement of horses racing, a bustling beach with bright, colorful umbrellas, or the directness of a lightning bolt.

All people have both yin and yang aspects within themselves, and the same is true for buildings and rooms. When these energies are balanced appropriately for the room, you can feel the harmony.

How do these energies relate to living or working spaces?

Creating yin energy is as simple as using curves, dark and soothing colors, and objects such as a soft flowing water fountain. To bring this relaxing energy into a space, try using round tables, playing soft music, or adding paintings of a water feature or landscape. Emphasize yin energy in bedrooms and bathrooms to create a more relaxed, calming mood. To harmonize these spaces, add a few candles or artwork with a bit of red to bring forward a touch of yang energy. This will complement the yin features and balance the room.

Family rooms, living rooms, kitchens, and home offices are considered yang rooms because these rooms are typically vibrant and high-energy. Use angular lines, bold colors, and bright lights to bring in yang energy. You might also choose to place tall plants, carpet squares, or cheerful family photos. As with the yin rooms, be sure to create balance in your yang spaces by adding elements associated with yin.

Do you want to create a relaxing space, a lively one, or foster an energy that's between the two? Thinking about your intentions for the room before you get started will help you make the right decisions when designing the space.

I once remodeled a party room in a high-rise apartment building overlooking a famous lake nestled into the city of Minneapolis. No one in the building was using the room, yet the view was breathtaking. The room felt cold and lifeless—not a great atmosphere for a party room! When redesigning the space, I paid careful attention to balancing the yin and yang energy to create a soothing yet lively feel that would attract people to the room.

One of the ways I balanced yin and yang in the party room was by creating a curvy bar top (yin) with a vibrant red color (yang). The existing black brick worked well with both yin and yang energy since the angular shape of the brick called in yang while its black color called in yin. I hung lively colorful artwork on the brick walls that featured both yin and yang elements. For the floor, I selected carpeting with angular and curved designs, and I placed furniture on it that had a mix of angular and curved features.

Above all, I focused on creating balance and harmony in the space. Yin and yang played off each other, and neither energy overwhelmed the other. As a result, the room felt simultaneously lively and relaxed—both energies needed for a party room.

Months later, my assistant and I were invited to attend an event sponsored by General Mills—a company I had been working with to help educate employees on healthy living. At the event, we played a video that showcased some of our interior design work. The manager who had organized this event was thrilled when he noticed the remodeled party room in the video since he happened to live in that building. He approached me and enthusiastically described how busy and well-loved the party room is now and how the décor is bringing people together.

This story exemplifies the overwhelmingly positive effects of creating balance within a space as well as the need to keep intention and purpose top of mind while planning your design. Use the five elements and yin/yang energy as basic guiding principles. If you want a space to feel open and energizing, incorporate a variety of shapes and colors that work together. These principles may seem simple, but that's a good thing. Much of Feng Shui boils down to good, clean design.

Your Turn

Here is an exercise to help you to balance the five elements and yin/yang energy when planning your design:

1. **Take the time to consider which elements are more prevalent within yourself and which you may lack.**

   As mentioned earlier in this chapter, it is possible to take an online Feng Shui element personality test to help determine your prominent elements.

2. **Make a list of the rooms in your home.**

   Walk through each room and examine the elements that appear throughout that area. Under each listed room, answer the following questions:

   + Are all five elements represented in the room? If not, which ones appear and which ones are lacking?
   + Do you need to add more or less of an element to your environment to create balance?
   + Which yin and yang elements are present?
   + Do you need to add more or less yin or yang energy to your environment to create balance? If so, which energy is lacking?

3. **Take one action to improve balance.**

   Start small. If you notice something is off-kilter after walking through one of your rooms, think of ways you can correct the balance. If you have an overabundance of fire energy in one room, for example, how can you either reduce the presence of fire or increase the presence of other elements? Could you add a piece of artwork, swap your red throw pillows for ones that are a more cooling color, or add an object that represents water or earth? Make small, incremental changes and notice how you feel in the days that follow. Does the energy feel improved? Or do you need to continue adjusting the space?

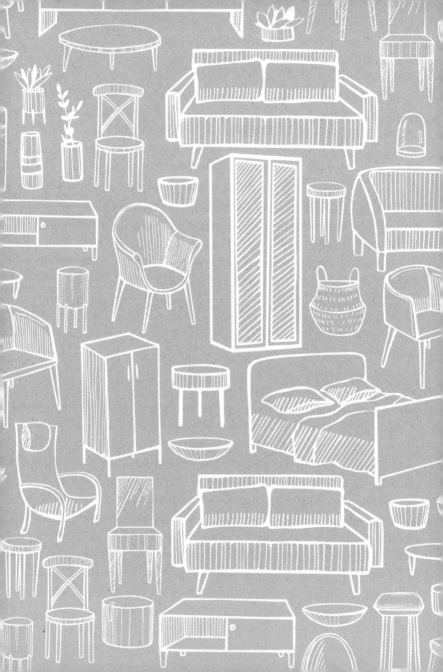

Chapter 5
Elevating Your Energy

Various factors can either elevate or dampen the energy of a space. Ultimately the goal is to raise the energetic vibration in your home or office so you feel better, your focus improves, and you gain mental clarity. In this chapter, we will discuss how to tune in to the energy of a room and address a few methods for elevating or improving that energy. But first, let's discuss one of the largest and most common energy drains: clutter.

Clutter, Revisited

We established in previous chapters that clutter drains us of energy, keeps us stuck in the past, and makes us feel uncomfortable. It prevents the flow of energy, hampers movement, and causes us to procrastinate. Clutter can also keep us socially isolated because we may be less likely to invite over our friends or organize family get-togethers.

One of my longtime clients, Ben, perfectly exemplifies the detriments of living a lifestyle defined by clutter. Ben is an energetic, successful businessman and my mentor in the multi-housing industry. I joke that he collects apartment buildings like he collects other valuables—cars, watches, artwork. Like many of us, he also collects magazines, thinking "one day" he'll have time to read them all. Meanwhile, they pile up in his office, causing clutter and distraction.

Once, Ben called me in a panic. One of his cars was lost. He owned forty vehicles at the time, which he had parked in different lots throughout the city, wherever he could rent a space. As you can imagine, it took much of his energy to keep track of them all. Ben loved his material possessions, but they were starting to take over his life.

Most of us don't have forty cars, but whether you own forty cars or four hundred tchotchkes, those items take effort to manage. Belongings can be a significant drain on your energy.

One day while working in one of his apartment buildings, Ben confided in me, "I'm exhausted from taking care of everything. I have no time for myself. All I want to do is fly off to an exotic island and stay there." He was so overwhelmed with his responsibilities and his many possessions; he wanted to run away from them.

Knowing I practice and teach Feng Shui, Ben called upon me to help. He didn't know much about the subject, but he was aware of its association with calming the mind and creating a sense of serenity. When he asked for my advice, I shared with him how clutter can hold you back, drain your energy, and promote apprehension or unease.

I also explained that the more stuff you own, the more space and time is needed to manage it, which might involve fixing, moving, insuring, cleaning, or storing the stuff. This also applies to items already stored away in a closet, attic, basement, or storage space. If you want more time and energy, own less stuff. Decluttering will free you.

After thinking about what I said, Ben hired Metro Interiors to help him declutter and organize. As a result, Ben noted, "I have more freedom, clarity, and focus. I no longer live in a constant state of anxiety."

Over the years, Ben has reported back to me that he has initiated decluttering in other areas of his home and office by himself. Working with a professional got him started, and when he began to reap the benefits and gain control over his life, it propelled him to continue the process on his own. We joke that decluttering is a lot like losing weight and having to keep it off—it takes time, dedication, and willpower.

The less you own, the fewer things weigh on you. As you go through the decluttering process and look at each item, only keep things you love, use, and need. Let the rest go. Decluttering is the first step as you begin creating a space that will help you flourish.

Tuning In to Energy and Emotions

One thing we know for sure is that life is always changing. These changes are necessary to keep evolving. Something you valued in the past may not have the same meaning to you today. If you are proactive and update your surroundings according to your changing circumstances, perspectives, and needs, you will inevitably feel happier and more comfortable in your space. Recognizing your truth and expressing that within yourself and your environment is a joyful and freeing process.

The relationship you have with yourself and your space is intimately linked with energy. Low energy or blocked energy can be caused by negative or harmful feelings as well as a cluttered or neglected space. When practicing Feng Shui, it isn't enough to overhaul a room and clear out clutter. You must also strive for continuous self-improvement and growth. Part of that growth stems from becoming in tune with your emotions.

Take a look at the emotional scale chart below to see the range of emotions. The emotions toward the top of the chart, such as joy, appreciation, love, passion, and enthusiasm, are considered positive. These emotions vibrate at a higher frequency.

Now take a look at the emotions listed on the bottom of the chart, such as fear, grief, insecurity, jealousy, and hatred. These emotions largely have adverse effects on us, and they vibrate at a lower frequency.

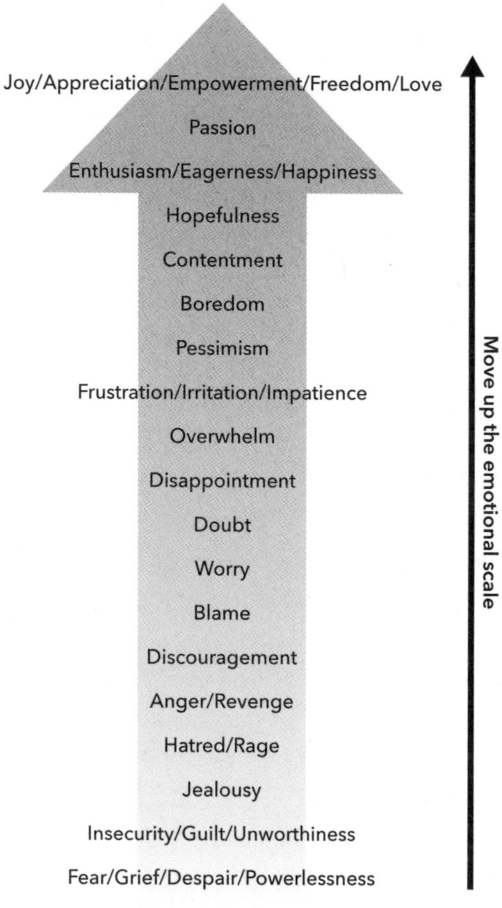

Joy/Appreciation/Empowerment/Freedom/Love

Passion

Enthusiasm/Eagerness/Happiness

Hopefulness

Contentment

Boredom

Pessimism

Frustration/Irritation/Impatience

Overwhelm

Disappointment

Doubt

Worry

Blame

Discouragement

Anger/Revenge

Hatred/Rage

Jealousy

Insecurity/Guilt/Unworthiness

Fear/Grief/Despair/Powerlessness

Move up the emotional scale

Figure 4: Emotional Scale Chart

All material possessions vibrate to a frequency that is associated with your emotions. For example, say you have kept a piece of art that was gifted to you by a former partner. The art is pleasant looking, but the relationship had been tumultuous and tense. Every time you look at the art, even though it may *seem* appealing on the surface, it evokes upsetting memories from that relationship. When you repeatedly relive those unpleasant events and feel the emotions on the lower end of the emotional guidance chart, you can easily fall into a state of depression, angst, or anxiety. You do not even have to look at the art for it to bring you down. If it is in your possession, it stays in your subconscious mind. On the other hand, when you choose to let go of the art, you let go of the negative emotions associated with it. Letting go can set you free.

The following statement on energy vibration (also referred to as chi, qi, or ki [Japanese]) within an environment is from the International Feng Shui Glossary: "Feng Shui concerns itself with the movement and containment of energy to create the most beneficial support for a person in their environment. The quality of energy is determined by its flow and the frequency of its vibration. By raising that frequency, we improve its quality and beneficial influence."[4]

We are all connected to the universe through energy. When our energy vibrates at higher frequencies, our positive

---

4. Ashdown, Prinzivalli, and Jampolsky, *The International Feng Shui Guild's Glossary of Universal Feng Shui Terms*, 22.

emotions, such as love, joy, and empowerment, increase. When that happens, we tend to attract more of the same energy, further amplifying these emotions.

The way to stay tuned in to higher frequency emotions is through your thoughts. If your thoughts are vivid and repeated often, they can become a reality. Positioning your furnishings with conscious intentions, using uplifting objects or artwork, and placing purposeful items will increase higher vibrations and elevate the comfort and peace you experience in your environment.

When I was married, my husband and I were at odds when it came to the upkeep of our home. He did not value well-organized and intentionally designed spaces, but that didn't stop me from continuing to organize and decorate. He would become upset with me for spending time and money on these types of tasks, which would bring down my mood.

In 2002 we moved to a new home with our three children. Shortly after the move, I became pregnant with our fourth. At this time, I was just finishing Feng Shui school and was becoming familiar with the attributes that either help or hinder a home. Our home was a spacious rambler in a beautiful neighborhood, yet it had some characteristics that were Feng Shui challenged.

As I became aware of the energy within myself and my connection to my environment, I also started to see disharmony between my husband and myself. We were not on the same page. I was working to raise my vibration through the intentional placement of our belongings and by keeping things in order. He did not support my efforts, and the more I tried, the more he created chaos. Life was becoming exhausting and unpleasant. Our priorities were different, as well as energetically incompatible. Through this disharmony, we eventually parted on a friendly basis, yet it was a difficult time.

Energy and Environments

After I moved, I realized many couples living on our new street had divorced. There are pockets of energy, even within neighborhoods that attract similar energy. After this experience, I always investigate many energetic and Feng Shui aspects of a home or neighborhood before renting or purchasing, and I encourage you to do the same. Before moving into a new home, try to learn about the situation of the person who is living there now. Why are they leaving? Did they lose their job? Are they ill? Are they moving on to better things? Or are they capitalizing on their successes and upgrading their living space? The energy footprint is established, and without intervention, it will likely continue to either positively or negatively affect the next person who moves in.

For example, if the seller is moving out because they earned a raise and are upgrading to a more expensive home, the overall vibrations in the home are likely positive. The person moving in is energetically set up to continue living in that energy and can gain similar successes. Keep in mind, it *is* possible to break a negative cycle and heal the space, but it does take time and effort to do so. If you are not willing or able to put in this work, I advise avoiding homes laden with negative energy.

Looking at these previous energy patterns (referred to as predecessor energy) can be true for anything you desire, whether it is living more peacefully, having children, finding a loving partnership, and so on. The more you find out about the current situation of the people selling their home, the more information you will have to guide your decision-making. If the energy is already moving in the direction of your dreams, that's a good sign.

Energy patterns exist in office and business spaces, too. I have noticed situations where the tenants in a particular part of the building keep changing. Each business in that seemingly "cursed" area keeps failing and eventually goes out of business. Making Feng Shui changes within the interior and/or exterior of a building is necessary to break this pattern. If you want your business to grow, look for an office space where the previous occupants moved out because they outgrew the space or were upgrading and expanding their company.

Aligning with Your Home

There are ways to change a space's energy positively through space-clearing techniques and making necessary Feng Shui adjustments, but it is an uphill battle when there are too many challenges to get the space flowing. I recommend rooting your-self in your intentions and not settling for a space that doesn't feel right.

Rachel was the second realtor I hired during the process of finding my home in 2018. It was a seller's market that year and a difficult time to buy a home. The first realtor and her crew were not aligned with my philosophy, and I was having a difficult time finding or purchasing a home. I placed offers on three different homes, all of which were over the asking price. None of the offers were accepted. Each of these homes needed a fair amount of work to adjust the Feng Shui and de-sign. I sensed the realtors involved thought I was super picky and challenging with my criteria.

I realized it would be in my best interest to work with a re-altor that spoke my Feng Shui language, so I decided to change realtors. I called Rachel, who was also Feng Shui certified. She gave me an intensive interview and helped me set my inten-tions for my new home. I told Rachel I did not want the incon-venience and expense of doing a total makeover. My intention was to find a home that was updated, well taken care of, and still had room to add my special touches and details. I had too many projects in my own life, and I needed to prioritize my time. I didn't want to pay over the asking price and hoped the seller would split the closing cost so I could afford to do some decorating right away. The previous realtor did not believe I would find this arrangement in the market at that time, but Rachel listened to my intentions and took me seriously.

Together, we began viewing homes that seemed to align with my criteria. Having the ability to see what a home could transform into, I would ramble on about all the changes I would need to make to create a comfortable home. When this happened, Rachel calmly reminded me of my intentions and encouraged me to stick to them.

When I recall walking into the townhome I would eventually purchase, I remember the big smile that lit up my face. The home felt fresh, clean, and well maintained. The woman who owned it was a trained butler and maintained large estate properties. Clearly her professional fastidiousness also applied to her housekeeping. The space was beautiful, had a nice flow, and there were no major Feng Shui issues that could not be corrected with simple adjustments. It was a blank slate, and I was free to add my touches on my timeline. Most importantly, the energy sang! I could feel the positivity of this space and knew it would uplift and support me instead of dragging me down.

I ended up buying this home for the exact asking price, and the seller split the closing costs with me. Later, I discovered that four other people had attempted to buy this property before I saw it. Each one had pulled out of the deal, even though it was the most beautiful home in my price range I had viewed. Although another woman attempted to put in an offer at the same time as me, she backed out because she did not want to participate in a price war. I believe that setting strong intentions held that home for me. It was just what I ordered.

Crucial Space Considerations

If you are seeking something or hoping to accomplish something specific, take the time to think about your objectives and write down your intentions. It does pay off. As covered earlier in this book, Feng Shui principles emphasize that intention is everything. And when it comes to purchasing a home, I advise you to consider using a Feng Shui–certified realtor. Check out the closest Feng Shui chapter or the International Feng Shui Guild's website to find certified realtors in your area.

When you're hoping to purchase or rent a new home or office, it is important to consider the energy of the space. To help you examine its energy footprint, I have made a list of nine crucial questions to ask yourself when seeking a new home/office:

1. **Who are the current occupants, and why are they leaving?**
   Learning more about a home's predecessor energy can help determine what kind of energy is lingering in the space.

2. **What is in the center of the space?**

The center represents your physical, mental, spiritual, or emotional health. In a business, it can represent the health of the company. When an area feels constricted or a bathroom or kitchen is in the physical center of a home, this can drain vital energy.

Solution: If there is a bathroom or kitchen in the center of the space, you can use drain stoppers and keep toilet seats down to prevent the draining of energy. Consider painting these areas earth tones, such as yellow, brown, rust, and orange. Accentuate with earth elements, such as beautiful stones and ceramics.

3. **Are there potential poison arrows?**

Poison arrows are sharp angles that can significantly hinder the flow of chi and create a negative energy force. They can create irritation and threaten your health. One example of a poison arrow is the corner of a wall jutting out and pointing to where you spend a good portion of your time, such as an area where you watch TV, eat, work, or sleep. Take a look at your home to see if corners are pointing to these areas.

Solution: Attach a round-faceted crystal to a nine-inch length of red string or fishing wire and hang it from the ceiling directly in front of the corner that creates the poison arrow. A round crystal breaks up energy's harshness, thereby calming the area and softening the energy. Crystals can also divert negative energy through refraction. Alternatively, you could place a healthy plant in front of the challenging area to block the negative energy from the poison arrow corner.

4. **Are the spaces conducive to activities that are important to you?**

   Think outside of the box when looking at the rooms of a potential new home or office. Can they be arranged or designed to serve different functions or support multiple activities? Can a storage room turn into an office or a bedroom turn into an all-in-one TV, yoga, and guest room?

5. **Are there angled doors, arguing doors, or piercing doors?**

   Doors represent the voice of the adult; their presence is linked to the adults of a household or, in the case of a workplace, to the owners of a business. Windows, on the other hand, are linked to children, innovation, and creative energy. Doors installed at an angle can be confusing and give you a sense of feeling "off."

Angled doors are auspicious in business but not for residential homes. Arguing doors occur when two doors bang into each other when they are open, which can induce arguments. Piercing doors describe a situation in which a home has three doors in a row through which occupants can walk in a straight line. This arrangement can cause heart problems, headaches, and can lead to conflicts in the home.

Solution: If you have an interior door within the home that is angled, you can balance and calm the energy with a round-faceted crystal hung from the ceiling with a nine-inch length of red string or fishing wire. Another option is to place a round rug in front of the door, either inside or outside the room.

To adjust arguing doors, convert one into a pocket or sliding door. If this is not feasible, you can also use the round faceted crystal adjustment between the doors as previously described.

To correct piercing doors, you should also hang a round-faceted crystal from the ceiling between doorways.

6. **Are any pieces of the Feng Shui Bagua missing?**

   A Feng Shui Bagua is a map used to lay over a blueprint of your space, which divides it into nine distinct sections.

   Solution: Please see chapter 8 to learn more about the Bagua and missing pieces. It is possible to correct missing pieces, but if they occur in a living room or other essential area, it may be a major undertaking. In these cases, the home or office may not be the right fit for you.

7. **Is the kitchen in the front of the home and seen from the front door?**

   A kitchen in the front of the house can cause eating and digestive disorders and make you think about eating and snacking the minute you walk through the door. Entering your kitchen through a garage door applies as well.

   Solution: If the kitchen is in view when walking through the door, try setting up a decorative screen as a buffer, if the room allows. If this is not possible, try adding a few taller plants or decorative items to create a barrier. Another option is to hang a round-faceted crystal between the door and kitchen to calm the energy.

8. **Is there enough storage?**

   Adequate storage space can help keep a home neat, organized, and clutter free. Bear in mind, it is best to only store items you still use but not on a daily basis.

   Solution: Use creative storage solutions (use vertical space, add shelving, utilize well-labeled tubs) or consider letting go of any object you have not used in a couple of years (try using the paper bag method described in chapter 1).

9. **How many immediate updates are required?**

   Will you need to make changes right away to feel comfortable in the space? Will your budget allow you to make them right away? If you cannot make the necessary updates soon, consider moving on in your hunt for a new space.

When making any of the adjustments mentioned in the prior list, it is essential to set your goals with a clear head and pure intentions. Never adjust when you are tired, angry, or hungry. Work on centering yourself through exercises, such as meditation or deep breathing.

Your state of mind has the power to change the vibration of the energy in your space. Let go and be open to how your changes come about. There is no need to control the results. Trying to control can hinder your solution.

Space Clearing

If you're decluttering your space or moving into a new one, try using a simple space-clearing technique to eliminate any lingering, stagnant energy. You can use any number of these techniques when you're feeling stuck in an area of your life or are going through an emotionally trying time. Space clearing can assist in physical and emotional release and aid in relaxation.

Smoke cleansing is one approach to clearing space. To start, purchase a sage stick that is ethically harvested (it has been threatened by overharvesting recently). If you find the smell of sage is too overwhelming, try burning palo santo wood instead (also ethically harvested). Start by opening windows and doors to let fresh air inside. Then light the sage or palo santo wood stick and blow it out so the embers start to smoke. Hold a bowl under the smoldering stick so the ashes fall into it. You may have to light the stick several times throughout the process.

Starting at your front door, move clockwise throughout your space, stopping every few feet to let the smoke penetrate each area, including the corners of the rooms. Wait until the smoke is flowing straight up before you move on. As you do this, visualize your positive intentions, imagining all the negative and stuck energy melting away. Continue moving clockwise until you return to your front door.

Smoke cleansing is far from the only effective space-clearing technique. Others include intentionally using chimes, bells, singing bowls, candles, or Florida water. Florida water is a citrus-and-herb-infused cologne known for its healing and spiritual properties (it's potent, so I usually dilute it with a 3:1 ratio of water to Florida water). It may be sprayed in the air or dabbed on the skin to promote clarity, healing, and positive energy.

All of the techniques I listed can be combined when performing your clearing (although Florida water *is* flammable, so be mindful when using it around candles). You may want to invite supportive friends to help you. For example, while you are lighting the sage, one friend could work with chimes or bells. Space clearing can produce uplifting and enlightening energy in your home.

By using spiritual objectives and materials in tandem with set intentions and adopting the philosophy of "bring in, let go," we can prevent our spaces from being overrun by things. Cutting clutter and keeping only well-loved, often-used items can go a long way in elevating the energy of our material possessions and, thus, elevating our surrounding environments. Once you're free from clutter and have practiced intentional space clearing, you can now begin the decorating process to invite in even greater comfort and joy.

Your Turn

Let's apply what you've learned about energy flow, vibrations, and decluttering to your life. Try these three steps to get started:

1. **Consider each room.**

   Which areas in your home need decluttering?
   Walk from room to room and jot down your immediate observations and reactions. Do you see
   junk piled up on tables or in the corners? Does
   a particular room make you feel uneasy, anxious,
   or simply uninspired?

   Which room caused the strongest negative
   reaction? What about it made you react the way
   you did? Can you identify a connection between
   clutter and the way it's affecting your life?

2. **Focus on one room at a time.**

   Even if more than one area needs attention,
   focus on your greatest "problem room" for now,
   and start with decluttering. When going through
   each of your belongings, ask yourself: Do I need
   this? Do I use this? Do I love this? If you don't,
   let it go.

3. **Practice space clearing.**

   Then, use one or more of the space-clearing
   methods described in the last section. Ring bells,
   burn sage or palo santo wood, spray Florida water, light candles—whatever feels intuitively right
   to you. Remember: The most important part of
   space clearing is your intention.

Chapter 6
Design Features

Our homes are mirrors of our inner worlds. If they feel chaotic, we have no chance of finding a sense of harmony or restoring ourselves from the day's hectic pace. Instead, our homes should be calming and instantly shift our moods once we set foot in the door.

As we established earlier in the book, homes may breed chaotic energy through clutter or general disorganization. Decluttering and careful editing of décor, artwork, and furniture is key. If we accumulate too many things, they can visually distract us and vie for our attention.

Once you declutter, you can begin to add special touches to your home to create a calming, nurturing space. You might choose to incorporate softer features, such as candlelight, soothing colors, indulgent fabrics and rugs, or maybe even a water feature or relaxing music. Executing design changes in a balanced way is also essential so your home's energy doesn't feel off (uncomfortable) or too much (overwhelming).

In this chapter, we will address some of the key design components associated with Feng Shui, including color, artwork, and furniture placement. But first, it is important to understand why the furniture, objects, and artwork we place in our homes are important and how they are tied to our conscious and subconscious selves.

Homes and Higher Consciousness

Every object in our material world originates first in the non-material universe. Allow me to rephrase this vital concept. Any item that has materialized in our reality first originated in thought-form. From where do these thoughts arise? Are they from inside or outside of ourselves? After contemplating these questions through spiritual studies, I understand that ideas come from outside of ourselves and are translated, by us, into the physical world. In essence, every creation comes from the spiritual realm with us as the receivers or conduits to transform those thoughts into reality.

A second important concept that is foundational to Feng Shui is the difference between poverty consciousness and prosperity consciousness. Many of us do not believe we can have comfortable and luxurious furnishings for our homes. Somehow, we think we are not worthy of them, or we think we will never be able to afford them (an example of poverty consciousness). Others believe there is absolutely no limit to what they can have in life in terms of comforts or luxuries (prosperity consciousness).

Having comfortable and luxurious décor and furnishings does not always mean they are wildly expensive. Why is there a disconnect between our perception of luxury and the cost associated with that pleasure? These disparities are simply due to belief systems. We choose our thoughts, and our thoughts create our reality. Sometimes we need to look deeper into our belief systems and make a conscious effort to change *them*. Changing your belief system sounds like an immense undertaking, but it really begins with conscious thinking and mindfulness. A famous quote (first stated by American businessman Frank Outlaw) captures this idea perfectly: "Watch your thoughts, they become your words; watch your words, they become your actions; watch your actions, they become your habits; watch your habits, they become your character; watch your character, it becomes your destiny."[5]

Once you change your belief system and thoughts and begin adopting a prosperity mindset, you open yourself to possibilities and acknowledge that you are worthy of a home that is a comforting sanctuary visually, spiritually, and emotionally. Be forward- or future-thinking and do not dwell on "what is," but instead, think about the way you want things to be. Those redirected thoughts will transform and shape your new reality.

In the book *Personal Power Through Awareness*, author and spiritual leader Sanaya Roman shares a powerful statement about energy and the incredible link we all share with our living spaces:

---

5. O'Toole, "Watch Your Thoughts, They Become Words; Watch Your Words, They Become Actions."

Every object in your home and your home itself is charged with your thoughts and energy. Every time you look at your house and think, "This is too small; I do not like it," you send that energy into your house. It will be there to help bring you down. Every time you say, "What a wonderful place I live in, how fortunate I am to have this place," you make your home your friend and ally. Then, at times when you are not feeling good, you will find solace and comfort in your home. If you want to move to a better place, start by loving what you have.[6]

When you are appreciative and in tune with your space, you are in a proper frame of mind to begin making any necessary adjustments. Send loving thoughts into your home as you endeavor to make changes. You do, after all, still appreciate your space; you only want to raise its vibration and improve the energy flow. With each change you make, pause to appreciate the positive effects (or recognize when something feels off and needs further adjusting). By taking your time with adjustments, you allow your surroundings to transform naturally and you're more likely to recognize when a certain design choice did or did not work.

Design Choices for Your Space

In 2019 I considered moving my business into my home. In March of 2020, when COVID-19 hit, I took the opportunity

---

6. Roman, *Personal Power through Awareness*, 14–15.

to make that happen. I now had the time and I was able to cut back on other expenses, so I went full force forward without looking back. To make this transition, I digitized my resources, got rid of three-quarters of the stuff in my current office, and remodeled parts of my home to make accommodations. When bringing a business into your home, it is crucial to keep it separate from other areas of your life; otherwise, it can start to take over. In other words, make sure you have specific areas designated for your business.

I chose two areas in my home to devote to my work—a room on the lower level and an area on one side of my garage. The lower-level office serves as my administrative space, and the space in my garage holds my design resources and acts as a place where I can create and design. To help tie these areas together energetically, I painted them the same color, putting a soft light-vanilla color on the main walls with rich, golden areas behind the shelving units I purchased for resources and samples.

When we make conscious decisions about our intentions when remodeling or redecorating, we raise the vibration in a room, which changes the space and can change our lives. For example, painting your bedroom a restful color can promote a good night's sleep, which will influence how you function the following day. Additionally, adding sufficient lighting, choosing the right furnishings and artwork, and taking the time to organize the area to be efficient and effective are all ways to contribute to your well-being and happiness. Becoming mindful of your redesign possibilities and understanding what will work is a process and takes practice.

Color

One of the quickest ways to change a space's energy is through color. Color provides a natural starting point for redesigns since it is often the first aspect of a space your guests will notice. The emotional responses produced by color are tangible, so it is important to make intentional color choices.

As with any other aspect of home design, it is important to balance color usage within your space. This can be achieved by understanding how colors represent the five elements, as discussed in chapter 4. If you desire calmness, use a color associated with water, such as blue or black. If you need to feel more grounded, use colors associated with earth, such as brown or yellow. Using energetic fire colors, such as orange or yellow, in your kitchen or dining room can increase appetites and make your friends more talkative at the table. Try using works of art to add splashes color if you cannot paint the walls in your rental unit.

It's always best to choose colors that you love and invoke positive feelings. Choosing a color palette just because it is trendy may not serve you in the long run, although viewing the "in" colors each year may inspire you. You can find the "colors of the year" by searching your favorite paint company, such as Benjamin Moore or Sherwin-Williams.

You may also draw inspiration for color palettes from fabrics or works of art. Many times, I have started designing a room based on a fabric my client loved (perhaps they were enamored with the floral pattern, a bright color, a contemporary design, or a fabric that evoked a sense of nostalgia). We created our color palette from the colors in the fabric, even if the fabric itself played a minor role in the overall design (perhaps showing up in a throw pillow or lampshade). Regardless, a well-loved fabric can provide an excellent starting point for pulling out tones and shades that feel right. It is important to be aware that each fabric has an energy or feeling associated with it, and this can be different for each individual.

There is a lot to take into consideration when choosing a paint color, such as the amount of natural light coming into the space. If you wish to select a deeper tone for a dimly lit room, it may be best to adjust the color by making it a lighter shade. You can achieve this by asking your paint store to lighten your paint selection by a certain percentage or by referring to the paint deck to find a similar color in a lighter version. Another way to counteract the effects of dark paint in a room without much natural light is to add plenty of artificial lighting, such as recessed lights, ceiling fixtures, and lamps to brighten the space. The amount of light in a room is a crucial component when choosing paint colors.

What if you love a particular shade of green, yet you instinctively know it would be too bright for your walls?

Consider using bright green in accent pieces, such as a vase or piece of art, instead. Think about the wall color and how the contrast would make the bright green vase stand out. Imagine painting the walls a deep gray or an off-white hue. Either color choice would work depending on how you want the room to feel.

I created a home office in a lower-level room in my townhome that had initially been used for storage. The walls were painted a drab gray, and there were no windows in the room. I chose to paint the walls a soft light-vanilla color to lift the room's spirit and give me focus (see chapter 4 for information on how colors affect you). Lifting the spirit of a room also translates to lifting the occupant's spirit. Painting a room is also one way to clear the area of negative or stuck energy. It can be energizing.

Floor-to-ceiling cabinetry was built behind my desk, and I accented that wall in a different color. The color I chose for the accent was a rich golden yellow called Sunset in Italy, and it peaked through my open shelving. This color gives me a sense of the sun's warmth and sparks my sense of adventure.

Choosing colors with intention will help you achieve your desired results quickly and bring you into balance with your life's goals.

Color Your Living Areas

We tend to spend much of our time in family rooms, living rooms, dining rooms, and kitchens. How do you want these main living areas to feel? Do you want bright and bold colors like fire red or bold orange? Or do you want to keep the tones softer, using colors like soft turquoise or tender green? Bold yang colors will give more energy to a space and make it lively. Some people need this type of power to lift their energy, while others want to create a calmer, more peaceful feeling with softer yin colors.

Everybody is different and has individual needs. It is important to consider your individual needs and the needs of your family unit when selecting colors. For example, if one family member suffers from anxiety, soothing colors can be beneficial. If a person is prone to depression or lethargy, lively colors may help raise their energy to a happier, more energetic state. Bolder, more vibrant colors can help provide more energy to tackle chores or work tasks.

Most people naturally decorate with a balance of bold and soft colors in their rooms, which helps create an internal balance. You could, for example, paint a room's walls pale green while accenting it with artwork, fabrics, or accessories that are red, orange, or yellow.

Remember: during our lifetime, our energy levels are influenced by ever-changing circumstances. We need to occasionally reassess our color and design choices and make adjustments that are compatible with our current physical and mental state.

Furniture

Have you ever walked into a room that felt overcluttered? Perhaps it was so crowded with chairs and tables that walking across the room seemed like a chore. Or maybe the furniture seemed too large for the space. Conversely, have you ever walked into a room that felt cavernous and unwelcoming? In this scenario, the furniture might have been spaced far apart, making conversations difficult.

These examples demonstrate the power of furniture selection and placement. Furniture, like wall color, can transform the energy of a room. Certain furniture choices can complement a space and energize or uplift its occupants. Other choices might clog the space and dampen its energy. When thinking about how furniture fits in a certain area, it's important to consider placement, the size of the furniture, the furniture's appearance (in terms of color, shape, materials used), and how the occupants will interact with the furniture.

When placing furniture, one of the first considerations is the room's focal point. This is the area people will see when they walk into a room (or through an apartment's door). Will they be greeted by the back of a couch (an unwelcoming focal point)? Or will they see an inviting and colorful love seat nestled behind a tasteful coffee table made of high-quality wood? Try to adopt an outsider's perspective, and walk into a room with fresh eyes. Where does your gaze land? That's the area to tackle first.

Another key consideration is the room's immutable features. These are the aspects of a room that cannot easily change, such as the shape of the room, the placement of the windows, and the ceiling height. You might, for instance, assess the location of the windows and think about ways to work around them instead of blocking them. Keep in mind, a room's architectural features can act as the main focal point. A living room fireplace, for instance, is a natural focal point, and it often makes sense to arrange furniture around it (making sure nothing is blocking the fireplace and that pathways are clear for walking through the room). Work with the space's architectural features instead of against them. Use the room's unique qualities to guide your choices.

You'll also want to consider the room's flow. Is there a natural pathway through the room? Perhaps the room has two doors or entryways, one on either side. In this instance, it's a good idea to keep a clear avenue between these two doors since the occupants will likely walk between them. In addition to following a natural pathway, each room should have plenty of space to walk through. No one should have to worry about bumping their knees on tables or maneuvering around floor lamps.

Another key feature of any room is lighting. Lighting is tremendously important since it can have a direct (and sometimes immediate) effect on a person's mood. Consider how to take advantage of natural light by keeping windows open, using mirrors, or utilizing light colors, which reflect light. You'll also want to think about how different areas of the room are used and how to incorporate lighting accordingly. Overhead lighting can generally illuminate the space, but you may need to amplify your lighting in certain situations, such as in an office or in a kitchen's food prep area (which could be illuminated using under-cabinet lighting). Many rooms will have overhead lights, and it's a good idea to assess how inviting (or uninviting) they feel. If they are too harsh, you could install a dimmer switch or swap the light bulbs for a warmer color. If your ceiling is relatively low, it's a good idea to use recessed lighting or ceiling-mounted light fixtures, if possible, instead of drop lighting.

Additionally, placing floor lamps or tabletop lamps, adding accent lighting, or installing dimmer switches can create a certain mood in the room. For example, low lighting and colored accent lights can create a romantic or relaxed atmosphere. On the other hand, bright, cheerful lighting can increase energy and productivity. You can also use lights to add areas of interest or draw attention to a certain spot. Adding a floor lamp beside a piano naturally draws the eyes to that feature. Or, installing accent lights in a curio cabinet or trophy shelf can call attention to these items.

Other details to keep in mind are furniture color, patterns, textures, and materials used. As discussed in the color section of this chapter, colors can have a powerful effect on occupants.

Do not haphazardly select a room's color palette, but instead, be mindful of the distinct effects color can have on people. The same is true of patterns. Busy patterns, such as floral or animal prints, can be energizing and fun, but they can also overpower a room (especially a small room) and produce nervous energy if used in excess. Balance and moderation are key.

When distinct textures are incorporated into your design, the effect can be pleasing to the eye and to the touch. Mixing textures with fabrics, area rugs, wall finishes, and more is a fun way to add interest to a room. If a neutral color palette is used along with an array of different textures, it can give the space a contemporary look.

In terms of materials used, I recommend using high-quality materials that will not easily warp or break. Investing in quality furniture shows respect for your space and yourself, and this investment can pay for itself over time. Keep in mind, high-quality pieces may not always be the most expensive pieces available. It *is* possible to source furniture and accessories from budget-friendly shops. I also recommend selecting pieces that are free of chemicals and toxins (which I discuss in more detail in chapter 7).

Other furniture-related practices include placing a water fountain in the career area of your home or room (see chapter 8 to learn about how rooms and houses are divided into distinct areas). When placed with intention, a water feature will bring in wealth and help keep your career—a life path—flowing smoothly. You can also use rugs to create distinct areas in your space. Make sure the rug is appropriately sized—not too big *or* too small—and is a color and texture that you enjoy. I recommend placing furniture partially or fully on top of a rug to tie the furniture and rug together.

Above all, have fun with furniture placement and trust your instincts. If your initial design feels off, don't be afraid to rearrange or try something new. Be bold, take advantage of the natural flow of the space, and make choices that align with how the room is typically used.

Artwork

We place art in our spaces for many different reasons—for beauty, inspiration, or to make a statement about who we are or what we believe. With Feng Shui, the placement of art can go one step further and support our intentions and desires, whether we want to create a sense of harmony, attract more wealth, have more support in our careers, or enhance a relationship. Artwork can also help balance the five elements in a room.

Paintings and prints speak to different people in different ways. For instance, let's say you're looking for a piece of art to hang over your fireplace that represents water (a good idea if you want to bring balance and calm that specific area). To make the adjustment, you might choose an abstract print with soothing blue and green lines, or you might select an oil painting of a fish, or you might go the literal route and pick a photograph of a mountain lake. It's important to trust your intuition and select artwork that calls to you or has some kind of connection to you.

When decorating, you might choose a painting with sentimental value—a piece of art from a special trip or a photograph of a beloved location. Whatever artwork you pick, the important thing is that the artwork resonates with *you*. How does it make you feel? Does it bring to mind calm and tranquility? Does it make you energized and invigorated? Or does it make you feel dark, brooding, or anxious?

When I first moved into my apartment after getting divorced, I needed to use Feng Shui to boost my energy. I was starting a new life. I left with no furniture, only taking my favorite art and accessories. Low on resources and recovering emotionally, I knew art would be healing and inspiring for me at work and in my personal life. One piece of art I hung right away was a brightly colored painting that featured blooming flowers. This was one of the first pieces of art I had ever purchased. It had a lot of good energy and movement, and that was just what I needed in my life.

Soon, I started to feel uplifted—emotionally and financially. In a short time, I grew my business significantly and began to feel joy again. As a Feng Shui consultant, I have seen changes in myself and my clients as the result of placing inspiring artwork. Art is a powerful way to bring your intentions to life.

In 2016 I was hired to work with a committee in a residential multi-housing building, Nokomis Square Cooperative. The building was originally a junior high school that was converted into senior condos. Even though most of the common areas had been newly redesigned, the building's occupants felt that decorative elements were missing in the corridor hallways, and the bare walls made it seem like they were living in an institution. The hallways were bland, unappealing, and (for some) even depressing.

I began working with a committee called the Design Enhancement Work Group, and after a few meetings with me, the group decided to create art galleries along the hallways. We would do one hallway each year—a realistic goal since the building was composed of seven floors with long hallways.

The first year, we adorned the first floor with an array of artwork in a variety of subject matters and mediums. After that, we chose themes for the next six floors. Some of the themes included cinema and theater, water, and history. We selected images that would bring back meaningful memories, such as local and worldwide landmarks, as well as pieces that would simply bring a smile to the residents' faces or become a conversation piece. One resident remarked, "We're so glad you included the photograph of the Riverview Theater. My husband and I had our first date there."

As the projects progressed, I noticed the profound impact the art was having on the residents. Their common areas were feeling more comfortable and more like home, and their spirits were lifted.

Additionally, the artwork was bringing people together. One piece we selected for the main floor (placed at the end of the hallway, partially into the lobby) was a large tryptic collage of the Minneapolis skyline. It was an interesting, colorful, and eye-catching piece. Next to it, we attached a small key to the wall that listed the names of the buildings that appeared in the painting. One residence said, "Whenever a family member or a friend comes over, I take them to see the collage of the Minneapolis skyline. It becomes a conversation starter while we discover and reminisce about our favorite landmarks."

At Nokomis Square, we also painted a large wall in the elevator lobbies on every floor. The accent color is a soft, toned-down green. After adding the painted accent wall, many residents commented on how the enhanced space felt more inviting (and less institutional!). One resident told me she now sits and relaxes while waiting for the elevator. Adding the green accent color helped create a sense of calm and serenity in a space where before the occupants may have subconsciously felt anxiety or a rush to keep moving.

The outside world can sometimes seem anything but harmonious, and it often feels ruled by chaos. It can zap our energy and leave us drained. We need a place to retreat and rejuvenate. It is essential to pay special attention to how we design and maintain our homes to best serve us and our families. We live in a society where rushing is the norm, but we can consciously make changes in our environment to remind us that there is more to life and we can (and should) take the time to smell the roses and "just be."

Your Turn

How will you make efforts to create restorative space in your home? What design features have you already incorporated that make it a calming retreat, a place that serves you well? If certain areas of your home are making you feel anxious or stressed, I suggest making a list of those areas. Once you have your list, write down one or two changes you can make to foster either a calming or energetic space. Some relatively easy changes include decluttering, changing the paint color, moving around or letting go of old furniture or accessories, or adding a few fresh pieces.

To modify a given area with intentional design choices, consider the following reflection questions:

1. **Is the style of furniture, artwork, or colors reflective of who you are now or want to become?**

2. **Does your furniture fit the space?**
   Consider the room's natural flow and how your furniture is placed. Additionally, think about the

furniture's size and attributes (color, materials used, texture).

3. **Does the artwork in your home make a statement about your beliefs, or do you find it beautiful or inspirational?**

4. **Do your color choices reflect you?**
   Do you love the color blue (for example), but have no rooms in your home painted this color? Perhaps your walls are yellow, but yellow is a color you dislike. This personal color preference can subconsciously make you feel uncomfortable or bring you down.

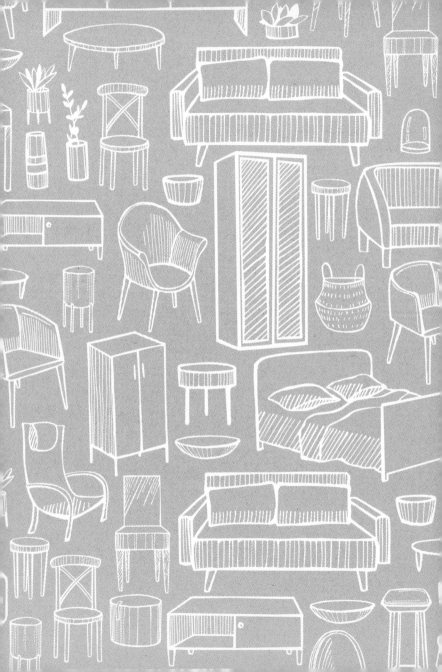

Chapter 7
Design by Nature

Imagine stepping into a room and being greeted by vivid flowers and the scent of green herbs. You hear the happy melody of songbirds, feel the warmth of a crackling fire, and are soothed by the sound of flowing water.

Biophilia, the love of life or living systems and the positive human response toward nature, is one concept I use to create feel-good spaces. This design philosophy draws inspiration from the natural world and adds vibrancy and vitality to indoor spaces by mimicking outdoor elements. Using biophilic principles elicits and inspires stronger attachments to the interior environment and helps calm your nerves—among other tangible health benefits.

I didn't know anything about biophilic design when I was a young child, but like many of us, I do remember finding peace and serenity when I spent time outdoors. Once, I stumbled upon the back of a semitruck not far from my home in a wooded area near the fairgrounds in Peoria, Illinois. One end of it was wide open to the natural environment, and my instinct was to create a little sanctuary inside.

I swept the uneven wood floor, brought in logs for chairs, and placed plants from the overgrown shrubbery of the small forest. Before I knew it, a few other kids from the neighbor-hood discovered my sanctuary and started to fill it with a few old or unused pieces of furniture from their homes. It became a peaceful shared space. When I learned about biophilic de-sign, it triggered the memory of the serenity I felt while sur-rounded by nature and actively bringing nature into the back of the old semitruck.

In these times, we have a greater need for biophilic de-sign than ever before. We're overworked, overstimulated, and bogged down by clutter (whether in our homes, our inboxes, or our own heads). As more and more people move to ur-ban or suburban environments, we lose the connection with nature that has always been a part of the human existence. Creating a sanctuary, whether indoors or outdoors, can offset some of our modern-day stressors. It creates and maintains positive mental, emotional, and physical health.

Biophilic design is based on the research of biologist Ed-ward Wilson, which dates back to the 1980s. Wilson asserted that humans have an intrinsic connection to life and nature and that when we are connected to the natural world, we feel good. It is in our biology. This profound connection with na-ture, he argued, should extend to our interior spaces.[7] I agree with Wilson's philosophies and have incorporated some bio-philic design into my interior design work. Though I am not

---

7. Rogers, "Biophilia Hypothesis."

an expert, the basic principles of this practice interweave naturally with Feng Shui and interior design.

In the decades since Wilson first popularized the term *biophilia*, biophilic design has steadily increased in popularity. More people are beginning to see the wisdom in reconnecting with the natural world, and medical professionals are identifying numerous health benefits associated with biophilic design. Among the benefits are increased mental alertness, reduced anxiety, decreased air pollution (when using living plants), and lower heart rate and blood pressure. A global study discovered that employees are far more productive and creative when working in an environment that incorporates biophilic design.[8] The list goes on. We are only beginning to understand the wide-ranging benefits of imitating nature in interior spaces, and each year brings us new research to support what many of us already intuitively know: people thrive when surrounded by soothing elements that invoke the natural world.

How Is Biophilic Design Connected to Feng Shui?

In many ways, biophilic design is a natural complement to Feng Shui. Although Feng Shui is more driven by intuition, symbolism, and tradition than biophilic design, both practices recognize the importance of harmony and the benefits of

---

8. Malik, "Plants in Offices Increase Happiness and Productivity," *Guardian*.

incorporating natural elements into living or working spaces. Additionally, both practices pay close attention to the surrounding environment and blend it into the overall design, utilizing factors such as sunlight, surrounding vegetation, topography, or the building's flow. When it comes to balance, both Feng Shui and biophilic design tend to use an assortment of complementary colors, textures, and shapes to create the rich variations we might find in a natural landscape. This is the embodiment of the yin and yang principle in addition to the five natural elements (wood, water, earth, metal, and fire).

Though they are similar in many ways, biophilic design and Feng Shui do have their differences. Feng Shui is more mindful of symbolism and chi, while biophilic design does not usually take these elements into account. For instance, a biophilic designer might not recognize the symbolic protection a backyard hill or mountain offers, or they might gloss over the potential pitfalls of having a downward sloping yard. A Feng Shui consultant, on the other hand, would recognize that a yard sloping away from the home can potentially drain positive energy (relating to health, finances, and more) and leave the home and its occupants vulnerable. To counteract the negative effects of a downward slope, a Feng Shui consultant might make adjustments to the space, such as building a retaining wall or intentionally placing specific elements to correct the problem (planting a tall tree, for instance, to heighten the chi or burying crystals with the tips pointing upward to counteract energy flow). When you choose to combine biophilic design with Feng Shui practices, you get the best of both worlds. I have found that these two methodologies can restore balance and add a sense of calm and serenity to a space—truly a match made in heaven!

Getting Started

You can easily add beneficial visual connections to nature in your own home. For example, you can use plants (including green walls or an herb garden), hang artwork that depicts nature scenes, or incorporate flowing water. All of these elements add to the feeling of returning to a sanctuary after a busy day in the world. Keep in mind that incorporating biophilic design into your space does not have to be expensive. It can be achieved through simple adjustments or additions—purchasing fresh herbs to grow in your kitchen, buying a giclée print rather than original artwork, or adding a modest tabletop water feature.

The Power of Plants

One simple way to reap the benefits of bringing nature into your home or building is to add houseplants, which reduce stress, support focus, and boost immunity. Even in dreary winter months, adding plants will be sure to brighten the spirit. You can place succulents on windowsills where there is plenty of light. During the winter months, they need very little water and are easy to maintain. Ponytail palms are resilient and add flair to a space. Other low-maintenance indoor plants to consider are Chinese evergreens, ZZ plants, aloe, bamboo, jade plants, and maidenhair ferns.

Plants do not have to take up a lot of space. Grouping plants in one area of a room gives the feeling of a habitat, which makes one feel as if it's a good place to be. Consider placing one large plant with a smaller plant draping over the sides in the same pot. Or adorn a console with plants on either side.

If you don't want to take care of real plants, the next best thing is using faux plants, although there is a difference in the quality of these artificial plants. Look for latex or silk and avoid plastic or dried. Quality latex or silk plants can embody a lifelike quality. A Feng Shui rule is to limit dried flowers and greenery because they are considered dead energy and can be a drain on your space. If something is a drain on your space, it can drain your energy. If your dried flowers have special meaning for you, listen to what your heart says about keeping them. Are they bringing you joy or pulling you down? If arranging florals is not your thing, try working with a trained floral designer who can bring finesse to your arrangements.

Natural Shapes and Materials

Organic forms can be captivating and comforting, and it is a good idea to use these naturally occurring shapes in fabrics, carpeting, wall coverings, sculptures, and furniture details.

Think of the winding flow of a river or the graceful curvature of an egg (although organic forms do not need to be literal representations). Together, organic forms and geometric shapes help create balance.

Biophilic design practitioners have identified several different areas or "patterns" that contribute to their designs, including visual representations of nature, nonvisual representations (sounds, scents, etc.), the presence of water (whether symbolic or actual), textures or contours that evoke nature (such as wood grain or flower petals), and plenty of open space/flow—just to name a few. As you can see, a symbol can be just as potent as an actual representation. You don't need to fill your home with plants and rocks (although you could!) to foster a relationship with nature. Instead, you could select a patterned rug that is reminiscent of river stones or purchase a piece of abstract artwork that reminds you of a blue sky over a yellow field of wheat.

Keep in mind, natural materials have greater restorative qualities than synthetic ones as they create a calming effect with their richness, authenticity, and stimulating textures. Choose natural materials, such as wood, stone, fossil, cork, and bamboo, for surfaces, flooring, and furniture. Accent rooms with these materials through accessories and artwork.

Light, Water, Air, and Other Considerations

Another important design element to consider is lighting. Good lighting is imperative for a comfortable and inviting space. The patterns created by sunlight and moonlight can evoke drama or instill peacefulness. If you are building a new structure or remodeling, plan and create an architectural blueprint where daylight comes in at angles or dappled sunlight filters through the windows, reminding you of the path of the sun. If your home does not have very much natural light, consider adding fixtures and light bulbs with different intensities and color temperatures. Candles and fireplaces can also add a soothing ambience. Other options include ambient lighting diffused on the wall, accent lighting, and dimming controls, which can all serve as stand-ins for natural light.

When designing a space, also keep in mind our natural inclination to seek safety and comfort. We tend to feel safer when we're protected by a structure behind us or overhead— think of a wingback chair, a reading nook, or a bay window seat. Create small spaces within larger ones by adding nooks with overhead trellises or lowered ceilings or consider adding recessed seating to offer a sense of protection. Elements such as these can reduce boredom, irritation, and fatigue, especially when their lighting is dimmer than that of the greater space surrounding them. These spaces create a cozy retreat where you can find solitude and comfort.

Adding a water feature to a room helps to reduce stress, stimulate and improve memory, and nurture concentration. Consider constructing a waterfall, fountain, or aquarium, but make certain the water remains clean and unpolluted. The imagery of water portrayed in art or the mere suggestion of water in a wall covering can work as well. The sound of running water can not only be relaxing, but it can drown out other external noises, such as traffic or the sound of barking dogs. In Feng Shui, adding a water feature to the front of a home or building can attract wealth and abundance and keep the energy flowing.

Nature is always moving, growing, and adapting, yet many interiors feel static and predictable. The air is stagnant, for example, and we may hear the same continual sounds, such as the ticking of a clock. We spend time staring at our computer screens and televisions, which can cause visual discomfort and headaches. Looking away from these devices every twenty minutes helps restore eye comfort and also produces psychological benefits. Introduce nonrhythmic stimuli, such as nature sounds, mechanically delivered breezes, and scents, to bring a sense of movement into your space and help you feel immersed in nature. You might consider adding an herb garden to a community room or your kitchen for the aroma. Building these elements into an interior environment is stimulating and helps the people living and working there feel happier and more alive.

Other alternatives to bringing the outside in is to strategically place a mirror to reflect an outdoor tree, garden, or lake. You could also incorporate nature-inspired art or use drapery panels to frame a window with a view. Painting the walls a deep, neutral color that contrasts with the exterior view is another way to accent the beauty of the outdoors.

Utilizing Rocks and Minerals

Adding rocks and minerals to your space is another effective way to incorporate biophilic design. You may choose to intentionally place gemstones or minerals in a room to create balance or invite new opportunities. Many Feng Shui consultants, myself included, use stones to correct imbalances, open new pathways, or welcome certain energies into a space. Rose quartz can foster love and bolster relationships. Purple amethyst has calming and purification qualities and can aid in overcoming addictions. Jade is an auspicious stone that invites luck and vitality.

Stones can be used as accessories (decoration that fits with the space), adjustments (to encourage or persuade a desired result), or materials. You might choose a quartz or granite countertop, for example, to infuse a room with the grounding energy of rock or citrine to call in more wealth.

There is power in stones. From Stonehenge to Easter Island, our ancestors understood the immense possibilities locked away in minerals and crystals. If you are still trying to gain an understanding of stones and their innate energy, I encourage you to try holding one and connecting with its energy. Notice the stone's weight, turn it over in your hand, and feel the energy coursing through it. Open your heart and listen to what the stone has to say. Does the energy feel grounding? Ethereal? Comforting? You might be amazed by what a simple mineral can convey.

I have personally witnessed the potency of stones many times in my life. Certain stones tug at me in a way I can't explain; I have learned to follow this pull and trust that the stone is either calling to me or to someone with whom I'm connected.

Recently, I wandered into a rock and gemstone shop in Arizona after I noticed a gorgeous piece of turquoise in the storefront. In the shop, I thought I might pick up a gift for one of my clients, a woman who had just gone through a divorce and was seeking a fresh start. While I was browsing, the shop owner approached me, carrying a white stone in her hand.

"I'm not sure why," the woman said, "but I was drawn to pick up this white calcite and bring it over to you."

At the time, I was looking at a different stone in the shop, but I was immediately attracted to the energy of the white calcite.

"I'm actually looking for a gift," I told the shop owner. "It's for a woman who is recently divorced and looking to make some changes in her life."

The shop owner's jaw dropped. "That's incredible," she said. "White calcite is the stone of new beginnings."

I stared in awe. The calcite represented the *very thing* my client needed most—a fresh start. The mineral had called to the shop owner, and she had answered.

Much has been written about the inherent power of minerals—too much to include in this volume. If you're interested in learning about the specific energies of certain stones, I encourage you to do a little independent research. I've included some relevant books in the recommended reading section at the end of this book.

Intuition and Nature-Related Symbols

Though Feng Shui is rooted in tradition and specific methodologies, it's a good idea to be flexible and trust your instincts, including when you decide to place nature-related symbols in the home. Many people are afraid to open themselves up and trust their instincts. It takes a certain amount of vulnerability, and it can feel strange at first (especially if you tend to be a "left brain" thinker). Even so, it's possible to start small. For me, "starting small" is embodied by a symbol from nature: the four-leaf clover.

For as long as I can remember, four-leaf clovers have played a role in my life. I tend to find them regularly—when I'm out for a run, strolling along the sidewalk, or simply in a friend's backyard. When I'm in need of a little extra luck, I ask for four-leaf clovers, and they come to me. I'll feel a tug of energy, look down, and see one. This has happened often enough that I know it isn't coincidence. It's energy.

When I find four-leaf clovers, incredible things tend to happen in my life. I distinctly remember finding one right before I purchased my first home and finding another during my son's high school graduation. One year, when I was going through a particularly rough patch, I would find clovers with *five* or even *six* leaves. They were potent representations of the extra support and luck I needed that year.

I believe one of the reasons these auspicious symbols appear is because I've created a literal and metaphorical space for them in my life. I have a special, tiny vase in my house where I place my latest four-leaf clover—I don't press it between the pages of a book or let it dry on the countertop. Instead, I honor it for a little while and let it go once it begins to wither.

One of my friends was in need of a little extra luck and approached me about finding four-leaf clovers. I advised her to prepare a space to welcome them into her life. As we were talking together, something in her yard caught my eye: a four-leaf clover. "There you have it," I said. "If you open yourself to possibilities, they will come."

A short time later, that same friend called me on the phone. "I found one!" she said excitedly. "I finally found one."

After this experience, my friend was more interested than ever in finding four-leaf clovers. She started to think about clovers as soon as the grass turned green and prepared a decorative vase for receiving them. Within two weeks of starting her manifestation practice, seven four-leaf clovers and two five-leaf clovers came to her without her even searching for them.

I am happy for the abundance of luck entering her life, and I understand that this is no coincidence. As with all things in life, you must trust your intuition and open yourself to possibilities. The same lesson applies to biophilic design. Let nature speak to you, as it has to me through four-leaf clovers. By bringing this piece of nature into my home and displaying it thoughtfully, I tend to conjure good feelings and usher in good luck (it's almost magical!). If you make an earnest effort to trust yourself and attract certain opportunities and energies to your life, they will come.

Your Turn

Though biophilic design is multifaceted and can involve many different elements, it is possible to dabble in it on your own. Follow some of the guidelines in this chapter (regarding lighting, color, water, plants, artwork, etc.) and, of course, trust your instincts. To get started, begin by reflecting on the following:

1. **Consider the environment in which you live.**
   Are you in an urban setting? Are you surrounded by trees? What are the sounds you hear throughout the day? What do you smell? Reacquainting yourself with your space is an important part of biophilic design. Only when you have an understanding of what you'd like to emphasize (more sunlight, better views of the trees, etc.) and how you'd like to correct (muting

street noise with the sound of flowing water or birdsong, painting walls in soothing earth tones, adding vitality to stale air with houseplants or air purifiers, etc.) can you truly begin to harmonize your space with biophilic elements.

2. **Look at the artwork around your home.**
   Does it still hold the same meaning as it did in the past? Is it still bringing you peace? Or is it time to introduce other artwork—perhaps pieces of art that incorporate depictions of the natural world or patterns that evoke water, trees, or a landscape?

3. **Reflect on your favorite natural elements.**
   What makes you feel most at peace? What energizes you? Conversely, what causes stress or unease? For instance, some people might find fire to be relaxing and nostalgic, while others may find that it prompts fear or nervousness. When you determine which elements are soothing, grounding, or energizing to you, you'll be better equipped to design your space accordingly.

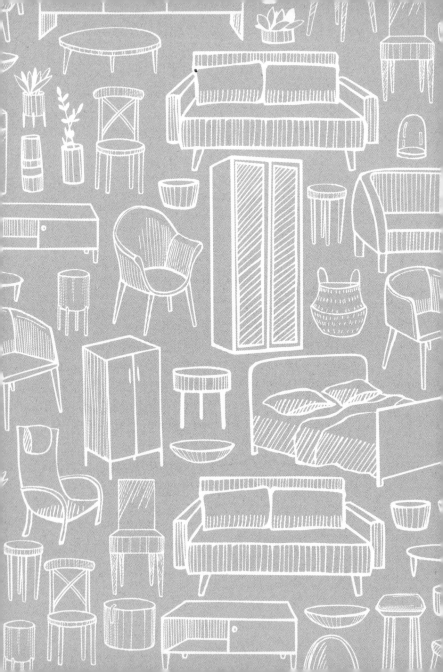

Chapter 8
Bagua Basics

After my divorce, I decided to start over when it came to furnishing my new home. I brought very little with me so I could surround myself with fresh new ideas and the things that mattered most to me. If you have ever been through a divorce or know someone who has, you know financial and emotional hardship usually comes with it, and I was no exception. It was important that my new space would support me in these two areas. With this in mind, I began seeking new accommodations. By then, I was very familiar with using the Feng Shui Bagua, a map that corresponds to different life areas that can be laid over the blueprint of a space. Having this knowledge and understanding how to use the Bagua helped me choose a space that fit my particular needs rather than a space that would pull me down or hinder my efforts.

A Bagua map is a grid composed of nine distinct areas, each corresponding to a specific life energy that can be found in your home. When selecting my new living space, I chose an apartment that had a larger wealth area that jutted out from the main floor plan. This type of area is known as an "extension" and can give the occupant(s) extra energy and blessings.

Instead of going out and buying all the furniture I needed, I decided to prioritize investing in artwork. I could not do everything on my limited budget, and to me, art is the soul of a room and can be inspirational. When I am inspired, I do better work and am more prosperous. I intentionally purchased a piece of art for my new apartment's wealth corner that had vibrant, abstract flowers in tones of red, purple, yellow, and apple green. The energy of the brushstrokes, colors, and flowers jumping out of the vase exuded abundance and joy. My intention in placing it there was to joyfully create more wealth and abundance so I could purchase everything I needed to set up my new home. That year, my business quadrupled! I was able to furnish my apartment as I liked, and more. I was even hired to redesign all twenty hallways in my apartment complex, which was an incredible opportunity for me and allowed me to feel even more at home in my new space.

Introducing the Bagua

In every home there is a story about the occupants that plays out within the décor and layout of the space. Mapping out the Feng Shui Bagua helps you clearly see your story and, therefore, where you might want to make adjustments or enhancements—not only physical adjustments but changes in your thinking process as well. Working with the Bagua is another way to make changes that can alter your life in the direction you choose.

When I get to know a client and their space, I can see what is potentially flourishing in their life and what is being challenged just by studying the way their floor plan interacts with the Bagua. With this information, in addition to discussing my client's experience and needs, I can determine which Feng Shui cure or interior design change would be appropriate in terms of creating a sense of wholeness and prosperity.

Feng Shui may seem like magic to a lot of us, and the principles of the Bagua can be especially mysterious. But by using the Bagua to organize our rooms, we can fill these spaces with the energy we need to achieve our goals and intentions. An ancient Taoist practice, the tradition of Bagua involves connecting physical spaces with specific life aspects. According to the Bagua, each part of our home relates to a certain part of our lives, including our physical well-being, financial wealth, and the health of our friendships and relationships. To put it simply, the Bagua can be classified as a tool or a map that can be placed over the blueprint of your home to show you the life areas that correspond to each part of your home.

There are eight areas of the Bagua that revolve around a central point that represents health. These areas can be arranged in a three-by-three grid (with health in the center) and include wealth, fame, marriage and business partnerships, creativity and children, helpful people and travel, career, knowledge, and family. Each area is supported by specific colors and the five elements, which are discussed in chapter 4.

When combining interior design and Feng Shui, you can design your space in a very intentional way. By supporting the nine areas of the Bagua, you cultivate a positive flow of energy, or chi, within and to them. The Bagua can be a tool to help manifest your specific intentions. What changes would you like to see in your life? You can infuse the energy of your intentions into your space and activate the energy of a particular area for positive results.

To begin your journey using the Bagua, you will create a diagram divided into a grid of nine equal boxes and label them with each of the Bagua's nine life areas (please see figure 5). You will then lay this grid on your floor plan (this applies to both houses and apartments) with the bottom of the Bagua chart aligned with your front door (to see the Bagua chart laid over a floor plan, please see figure 6). In most cases, the front door, as shown in figure 5, will fall in the area of either skills and knowledge, career and life path, or helpful people and travel. Of course, there might be a few exceptions based on the layout of your home (see the section about extensions and missing pieces for more).

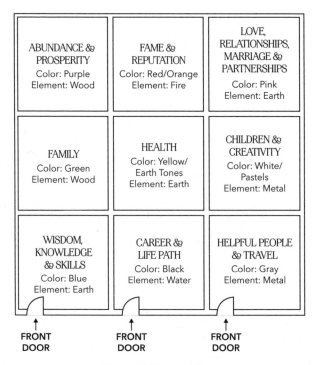

ABUNDANCE & PROSPERITY Color: Purple Element: Wood	FAME & REPUTATION Color: Red/Orange Element: Fire	LOVE, RELATIONSHIPS, MARRIAGE & PARTNERSHIPS Color: Pink Element: Earth
FAMILY Color: Green Element: Wood	HEALTH Color: Yellow/ Earth Tones Element: Earth	CHILDREN & CREATIVITY Color: White/ Pastels Element: Metal
WISDOM, KNOWLEDGE & SKILLS Color: Blue Element: Earth	CAREER & LIFE PATH Color: Black Element: Water	HELPFUL PEOPLE & TRAVEL Color: Gray Element: Metal

FRONT DOOR   FRONT DOOR   FRONT DOOR

Figure 5: Bagua Chart

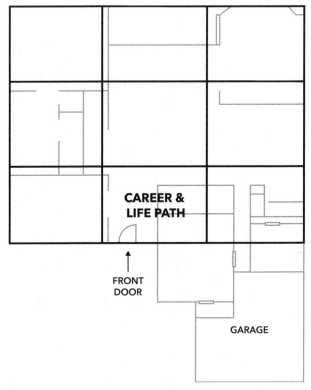

CAREER & LIFE PATH

FRONT DOOR

GARAGE

Figure 6: Orienting Bagua with Front Door

When you're adjusting your home to the Bagua, it is important to note that different levels need to be mapped separately. For an upper or lower level, the Bagua grid will be aligned with the walls and oriented to the direction of the staircase. However, when there is a short distance (say, three or four feet) to the wall from the top or bottom of a staircase, the orientation changes and the Bagua is rotated 180 degrees.

In this chapter, I focus on applying the Bagua to a house or apartment, but the Bagua can be used in any space—an office, a particular room, or even your desk. You need only orient the Bagua grid with the main entry point (for your desk, that means the place where you are seated) and proceed from there.

Once you have mapped out where each of the nine areas falls in your space, you can begin making adjustments or energizing specific areas. Since this process can be quite involved, I encourage you to only focus on one floor at a time. We will discuss each of the nine areas later in this chapter, and I will give examples of potential adjustments that can be made in each area, but first I want to address a particularly tricky aspect of floor plans: extensions and missing pieces.

Extensions and Missing Pieces

When you place your Bagua grid over a perfectly square or rectangular floor plan, it is fairly easy to divide your home into nine equal spaces. Many homes, however, are shaped irregularly. What then?

In Feng Shui practices, we refer to these floor plan irregularities as extensions (areas that extend off the main house) or missing pieces (parts of the square/rectangle that are absent). Extensions are considered a blessing and can bring you luck or expand your success in the corresponding areas. If, for example, your home has an extra room off the relationships and love area, that particular area has the potential to be especially potent. On the other hand, missing pieces can represent challenges or may cause a lack of energy in the corresponding areas. If your home has missing pieces, adjustments can be made to increase that area's energy and create balance.

It is possible for your front door to be placed inside a missing piece (see figure 9). If that's the case, the Bagua is aligned with outermost wall of your house and the front door is *behind* the bottom row of the Bagua grid (where the wisdom, career, and helpful people areas appear). Although the front door can be behind the Bagua's bottom row, it can never be in front of it. If the front door juts away from the rest of the house (as in figure 10), it creates a missing piece or pieces.

When considering whether or not your floor plan includes extensions or missing pieces, keep in mind that attached garages or screened-in porches are included in the Bagua—anything attached to your home that has a roof and sides. Attached decks are not included, since they do not have both a roof and sides.

Please see figures 7, 8, 9, and 10 for detailed illustrations and examples of extensions and missing pieces.

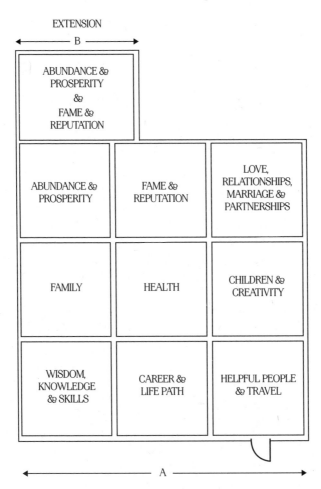

EXTENSION

B

ABUNDANCE & PROSPERITY & FAME & REPUTATION		
ABUNDANCE & PROSPERITY	FAME & REPUTATION	LOVE, RELATIONSHIPS, MARRIAGE & PARTNERSHIPS
FAMILY	HEALTH	CHILDREN & CREATIVITY
WISDOM, KNOWLEDGE & SKILLS	CAREER & LIFE PATH	HELPFUL PEOPLE & TRAVEL

A

Extensions are considered a blessing and can bring you luck or expand your success in a corresponding area.

Guidance: If the measurement of B is less than 1/2 of A, then an extension exists.

Figure 7: Example of Bagua Extensions

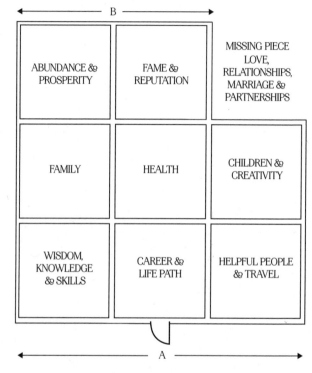

ABUNDANCE & PROSPERITY	FAME & REPUTATION	MISSING PIECE LOVE, RELATIONSHIPS, MARRIAGE & PARTNERSHIPS
FAMILY	HEALTH	CHILDREN & CREATIVITY
WISDOM, KNOWLEDGE & SKILLS	CAREER & LIFE PATH	HELPFUL PEOPLE & TRAVEL

Missing pieces can represent challenges or may cause a lack of energy in the corresponding area.

Guidance: If the measurement of B is greater than 1/2 of A, then a missing piece exists.

Figure 8: Example of Bagua Missing Pieces #1

The front door can be behind the Bagua map when
the home or building is shaped like the diagram
below. However, this does create a missing piece.

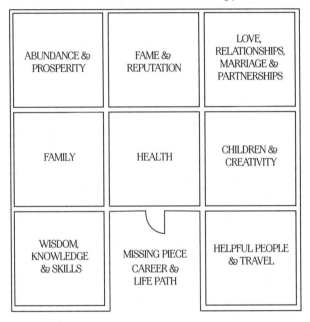

ABUNDANCE & PROSPERITY	FAME & REPUTATION	LOVE, RELATIONSHIPS, MARRIAGE & PARTNERSHIPS
FAMILY	HEALTH	CHILDREN & CREATIVITY
WISDOM, KNOWLEDGE & SKILLS	MISSING PIECE CAREER & LIFE PATH	HELPFUL PEOPLE & TRAVEL

Figure 9: Example of Bagua Missing Pieces #2

When a home or building is shaped like the diagram below, the front door can never be in front of the Bagua map. Therefore, it creates a missing piece or pieces.

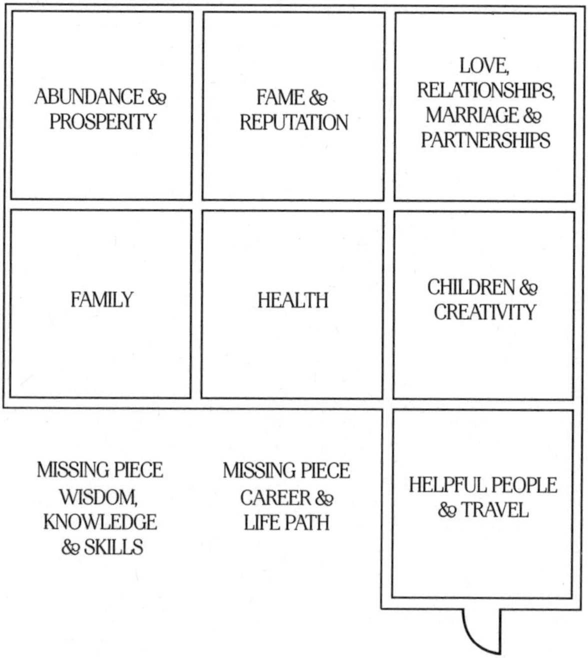

ABUNDANCE & PROSPERITY	FAME & REPUTATION	LOVE, RELATIONSHIPS, MARRIAGE & PARTNERSHIPS
FAMILY	HEALTH	CHILDREN & CREATIVITY
MISSING PIECE WISDOM, KNOWLEDGE & SKILLS	MISSING PIECE CAREER & LIFE PATH	HELPFUL PEOPLE & TRAVEL

Figure 10: Example of Bagua Missing Pieces #3

In my own life, I have experienced the blessings associated with extensions. When I was a young mother, I lived in a house with an attached garage that extended off the Bagua region correlating with helpful people and travel. At this time, I was busy running my own business *and* raising four young children, so I relied on assistance from both a wonderful nanny and a housekeeper. Life takes odd turns sometimes, and unfortunately, both had to quit around the same time. I was left with the momentous task of replacing two individuals that I had known and trusted for years.

I decided to tap into the energy of my home's garage extension to bring helpful people into my life. I was already planning to stage a boutique jewelry show and used this event as an opportunity to put my intention into the space as I was preparing. I called upon that extension to act as a catalyst to draw in a new nanny and a housekeeper, and I also rang a bell in the space to summon the help I needed.

That weekend, someone stopped by my jewelry display. As we were chatting, they asked out of the blue, "Do you need a nanny?"

I was flabbergasted. I told them that I was, in fact, searching for a new nanny and needed to hire someone as soon as possible. We were a perfect match.

But the story doesn't end there! Not long after they left, someone else showed up and began to peruse the jewelry selection. This person approached me and asked if I needed a housekeeper.

Again, I was stunned. I told them that I was, indeed, seeking a housekeeper. They informed me that one of their close friends worked in housekeeping and was looking for more work. And that's how I ended up finding my new housekeeper.

This sudden abundance of helpful people in my life was no coincidence. It was the direct result of me placing my intentions in the helpful people extension of my home and asking for these people to arrive.

Extensions have power and can provide incredible blessings, but what about missing pieces? When a space is lacking certain areas that correspond to the Bagua, an imbalance is created. Fortunately, these imbalances can be corrected. One way to create the illusion of a whole floor plan is to add a mirror that reflects into the missing area. For instance, if you're missing the wisdom, knowledge, and skills area of your floor plan, you could add a mirror to either the family area or the career and life path area, making sure the mirrors are hung on walls perpendicular to the missing piece and are facing into the room so the area feels extended. If adding a mirror doesn't fit with the room's aesthetic, you can always tuck a small mirror behind a painting to conceal it. Again, the important part of this action is *intention*.

When it comes to making adjustments, mirrors are a particularly versatile and potent tool for correcting Bagua imbalances. They may be used to guide the flow of chi, expand or amplify a particular space, or distort negative energy (convex or concave mirrors are particularly effective for this). One of my clients, a landlord, was hoping to rent one of his houses. He hired me to make the space more inviting by making a few adjustments. One of the last things we did was hang a mirror with the intention that the first person who viewed the home would rent it. My client embraced this action and wholeheartedly set his intention. Later, he called me and told me the good news: he had rented his house to the very first people who walked through the door.

Aside from mirrors, it is possible to compensate for missing pieces by modifying outdoor spaces so they align with the Bagua. You might plant a tree or a shrub or place a lawn ornament (a stone or statue, for instance) to represent the corner of the missing section. You might also use crystals to influence or redirect chi. Think of these objects as anchors to ground the space and make up for the missing piece.

Bagua Areas

Once you have determined where each Bagua area is located in your home, including extensions and missing pieces, the real work begins. You can now begin making adjustments and setting your intention to improve specific life areas.

Each of the nine regions of the Bagua are connected to specific elements and colors (as seen in figure 5). These can be incorporated into each space in creative ways. For instance, the career region is supported by the water element and the color black. You do not, however, have to literally place a water feature in this area or paint it black. Instead, you might choose to hang a piece of artwork that is reminiscent of water, intentionally place a piece of black onyx, or add an accent rug that features water-like waves.

You might even decide to *not* include the corresponding element in a specific Bagua region. Instead, you might choose to incorporate a *supporting* element. For instance, metal supports water (think of how a metal vessel can carry water), and you could include a representation of metal in the career region instead of a portrayal of water. When you're playing with elements, always do your research and proceed with caution. Some elements actively undermine other elements (earth absorbs water, for example). For more information about complementary (creation) elements—as well as clashing (destruction) elements—please refer to chapter 4.

In the same way you might play with elements, you can also get creative with color. If you're redoing your family section according to the Bagua, you are not obligated to paint that room green! Even though green is the corresponding color, you could represent it in subtle ways—perhaps placing a painting with some green accents on one of the walls or a family photograph that features green grass. Or you might choose to display a green vase or another decorative item in the room. Furthermore, you might select shades of green that are closer to blue (seafoam green, teal, mint), yellow (chartreuse, pear green), or brown/gray (olive green, sage). How you incorporate color is up to you. Do what feels right (using the Bagua as a guide) and, as always, trust your intuition.

As you're beginning to make adjustments in certain areas of your home, I encourage you to not overload or bog down the space with too many symbols or intentions. When areas are cluttered, it's more difficult for energy to flow freely. When it comes to the Bagua (and Feng Shui design, in general), less is more.

The following sections share the detailed meanings of each area of the Bagua as well as the color(s) and elements they represent. I also include ideas for integrating each element and color into the space. Keep in mind, these ideas are merely examples, and they may or may not suit your space or your style. It is important for you to feel comfortable and at peace in your home—or any space you regularly inhabit—and that's where your intuition and ingenuity comes into play. In short, use the following examples as inspiration, not strict guidelines.

Note: If there's a certain part of your life that needs a boost, you may want to focus on that particular area first. Additionally, if parts of your life are working well, leave those areas alone. There's no need to adjust what already feels right.

Wisdom, Knowledge, and Skills

Enhance and activate this area when you want to acquire new skills, increase your knowledge in areas that interest you, or work on self-cultivation and inner growth. The color represented in this region is blue, and the element is earth.

Idea

Consider incorporating a meditation space and/or library in this area of your home. If the space is not conducive to that, try a small-scale change such as intentionally placing a piece of pottery or a ceramic object (representative of earth) in the room.

Family

This area represents your immediate family as well as close groups of people you are associated with, such as companies, neighbors, faith organizations, and committees. Enhance and activate this area when you want to strengthen good relationships within any of these types of groups. The color represented in this area is green, and the element is wood.

Idea

This is an ideal place to create a family photo wall if the space allows. Or you could choose to add a plant, which embodies both the wood element and the color green.

Abundance and Prosperity

Enhance and activate this area when you want to attract money and material wealth. This area is not only for finances but for anything you desire in abundance. What would you like to have more of? Consider an abundance of opportunities, love, or friends. The color associated with this area is purple, and the element is wood.

Idea

Place houseplants or a carved wooden object in this area to represent wood and growth. Since water supports the growth of wood, you could opt to add a water feature instead, such as a water fountain or a photo or piece of art with a body of water represented. Or you could incorporate a black object (black represents the water element) to attract the flow of abundance.

Fame and Reputation

Enhance and activate this area when you want to shift your fame and reputation. What do you want to be recognized for? Do you want to become famous? This aspect of the Bagua is associated with how the world sees you, whether it pertains to your personal or professional life. The corresponding colors are red and orange, and the element is fire.

Idea

This is a good space for adding a fireplace or candles. You could also choose to place or hang awards in this region.

Love, Relationships, Marriage, and Partnerships

This area of the Bagua represents marriage, significant relationships, or business partnerships. Enhance this area when you want to improve and create stability within these types of relationships. You can also activate this area to "call in" or attract one of these partnerships. The corresponding color is pink, and the element is earth.

Idea

If you are trying to attract a love partnership, add art that illustrates or represents a couple. Make sure the art reflects the way you would want to feel with that partner. Add decorative gemstones, pottery, or ceramics to ground the energy and activate your desired intention.

Children and Creativity

This area represents the well-being of your children or your inner child, and it can also support couples who are trying to conceive. Additionally, this area is associated with creativity and can be used to spark your imagination, improve communication, and support new ideas and projects. The representative colors are white and pastels, and the element is metal.

Idea

Activate this area with playful artwork and lots of light. Consider placing metal sculptures to make this area a source of inspiration and originality.

Helpful People and Travel

This is the area you will want to activate when calling in people and benefactors who can help you. It is also the area to address when you want to travel and go on adventures as well as a space to adjust if you want to sell your home. The color to add here is gray (or silver), and the element is metal.

Idea

Add a bell or some chimes in this area to energetically call in the right person or group to help you in your endeavor. Hang photos of places you would like to visit, or if you prefer a more interactive piece, hang a large decorative map and track your travels with pushpins.

If you are trying to sell your home, write a note and leave it in this area, thanking your home for the time you spent in it and releasing it to its new owners. This allows you to fully let go of your home so the new occupants can comfortably settle in.

Career and Life Path

This area relates to using your abilities, talents, and interests, whether in your profession or everyday life. It is associated with your work and how you make your living. As a whole, this area reflects your life path and personal journey. The color for this area is black, and the element is water.

Idea

Place a water fountain or hang a photo or piece of art depicting water, such as a lake or ocean, to represent the flow of life. You can also add a mirror, which represents water in Feng Shui.

Health

Last but certainly not least is the center of the Bagua. This area is considered the most important as it represents physical, mental, emotional, and spiritual health. Without good health, all areas of your life are negatively affected, and it can be difficult to activate the other Bagua areas. Yellow and other earth tones represent this region, and the element is earth.

Idea

Consider adding a round, faceted crystal in the center of this area, using a nine-inch length of wire or string to hang it from the ceiling to calm the space. Add artwork with earth-toned colors as well as crystals and stones to activate this part of the Bagua. Healthy living symbols, such as fish, birds, and plants, can also be included.

The Three Secrets of Reinforcement

The way you choose to apply the Bagua to your space is entirely up to you. You can be as literal or as imaginative as you'd like with your interpretation of the guidelines. The most important part of the entire process is your intention. If you want to achieve your desired results, you must vocalize your intentions, and they must be authentic. It's difficult to make significant life changes if you're resistant to the energies that could help foster the change.

If you'd like to leverage the Bagua to assist you in a specific area, it's not enough to simply redecorate a room or add some paint. You have to focus on what you would like to bring into your life—the positive changes you'd like to see. To make your intentions clear and to tap into the energy of your space, I recommend starting with the three secrets of reinforcement.

Secret of the Body

When you are offering your intention, it is important to consider both your physical presence and how you place your object. Instead of slouching and crossing your arms over your body, stand tall and open your palms (or clasp your hands as if in prayer). Your stance should convey confidence, exude positive energy, and infuse the area with your mindfulness and purpose. Then you can place the object in an area that feels right to you.

Secret of the Mind

When setting your chosen object in the space, it is important to do so with intention. Your conscious intentions are tremendously important. Decide what you will place in your space and why. What meaning does the object or accent have to you? How does it relate to the Bagua?

Once you've answered those questions, take the time to visualize the end result. Don't just think about possibilities, but imagine your goals as if they have *already* happened. If you're hoping for a career change, picture yourself in your new role. If you'd like your health to improve, picture yourself healthy and thriving. Visualization is a powerful tool, and the more you believe in the end results, the more likely they will happen.

Secret of Speech

Lastly, bring forth your intention through speech. Stand in your space and recite the following mantra: Om Mani Padme Hum (pronounced OM MAH-nee POD-me HUM). The literal translation of this Sanskrit phrase is, "Praise to the jewel in the lotus," but the symbolic meaning is closer to, "Obtain enlightenment through following a pure path, built on wisdom and love."[9] Personally I associate this phrase with a lotus blossom opening to reveal its true essence, which is the soul. Regardless of your interpretation, it is a simple and beautiful sentiment that is meant to help you open yourself to possibilities after stating your intentions. Say this mantra nine times (an auspicious number in China) and release your intentions to the universe. By going through this ritual, you can free yourself from worry and stop fretting about the outcome of your stated desires.

Remember: Only make adjustments to a space when you are in a positive frame of mind. If you attempt these three reinforcement steps when you're feeling sullen or angry, that mood will be drawn into the room and become part of your intention.

---

9. Wangdu and O'Bannon, "What Could Mean More? Om Mani Padme Hum."

Your Turn

Now that you have a basic understanding of the Bagua, its associated elements and colors, and how to align the Bagua with your space, I encourage you to give it a try.

1. **If you're able, find a floor plan of your house and start mapping out your space using the Bagua map.**

   Is it easy to divide your home into nine equal parts? Or do you notice irregularities right away (either extensions or missing pieces)?

2. **If you're dealing with missing pieces, what are some adjustments you can make to correct the energy imbalance?**

3. **Focus on a specific area.**

   Once you've mapped out your space, take a look at the Bagua chart. Is there one particular area that calls to you? What parts of your life could use a blessing or an energy boost? Where would you like to focus your attention? If multiple areas are calling to you, pick one and center your intentions around it. Then, using the principles you've learned in this chapter, start making adjustments.

   Remember: Intention is key! Fill your space with focused positivity and *believe* that you are worthy of blessings and constructive change.

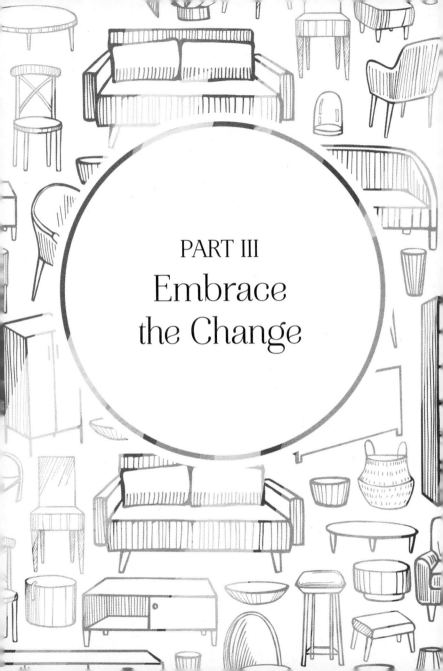

PART III
Embrace
the Change

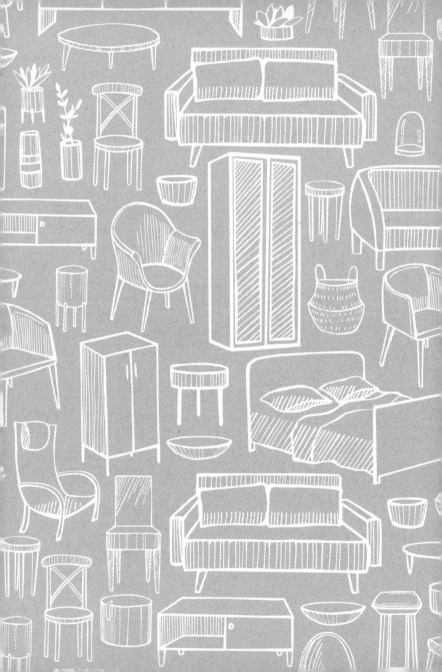

Chapter 9
Enhancing Your Healthy Environment

Your surroundings can have a profound impact on your personal health and well-being. The airflow and air quality in your home, the amount of sunlight that filters into your office, the materials you choose for your mattress and bedding—these factors (and many more) can affect your physical, mental, and emotional health. People sometimes say, "You are what you eat," when referring to dietary health. I would also add: "You are your surroundings."

Though creating healthy living and working spaces has always been important, it became even more relevant and urgent with the start of the COVID-19 pandemic. Not only were we attempting to avoid catching a nasty virus, but many of us were also suddenly confined to a small environment. Instead of regularly leaving the house to go to the office, eat dinner in a restaurant, or grab a cup of coffee with friends or colleagues, many of us were stuck at home. Life shifted, and we (and our environments) needed to adapt with it.

In my own life, I decided to use this opportunity to move my business into my home. I had been in my current office space for eleven years prior to the pandemic, but in the past two years, I sensed something was off. However, I delayed the decision to relocate my office to my home because I felt it would be viewed as unprofessional. I felt stuck and did nothing about it until COVID-19 emerged and life began to change dramatically for many people. My intuition immediately told me this was my opportunity to make some changes, and I decided to go forward and make arrangements to move my business into my home. I sensed this would be the new norm for many small business owners, and that, indeed, seems to be the case.

The process of relocating my office into my home was a journey that led me to increased clarity, focus, and direction in my business. Gradually the feeling of being stuck began to diminish. This process took six months and included decluttering, refining my focus on what to keep and what to let go, and remodeling my home. I knew I had to take one step at a time and plan deliberately because it was a lot to manage. The silver lining of COVID-19 for me was that it gave me the opportunity and time to make the necessary adjustments to achieve my goal. Contrary to my apprehension about moving, my business began to flow more smoothly and efficiently, and my profits started to increase.

During the same time period, I noticed several friends and family members making changes to their living and working spaces. Many people also decided to make intentional lifestyle changes to keep the virus at bay. Surprisingly these everyday modifications led to some unexpected blessings. Many gained clarity in their lives or discovered positive opportunities as a result of the crisis.

My sister commented that when almost everything was stripped from her socially and outwardly, she found out what was most important. She said that the changes made in their home were nurturing for her whole family, which includes a husband and six children. It brought them closer as they enjoyed activities together, such as planning and cooking meals. They knew the summer of 2020 was going to be different with the kids home (no summer school or other activities) and no gatherings with friends.

With the money they would have normally spent on summer school, my sister's family decided to invest in their home environment and create an outdoor living room on their deck. In the summer, their magnolia trees already acted as a natural barrier in front of their second-floor deck, creating privacy and beauty. They added a lovely outdoor sectional and a cocktail table, chairs with a floral print, and several potted plants. On the exterior wall, which was shared with their indoor living room, they added a shelf for accessories and weatherproof artwork. This became their private getaway and place of entertainment with the immediate family. Inspired by their revitalized outdoor space, my sister is now planning to change many other parts of her home to increase family enjoyment.

Though the COVID pandemic has been difficult in many ways, countless people (my sister and myself included) have used it as an opportunity to improve their living spaces. However, I believe that creating and enhancing healthy environments should always be a priority, pandemic or not. Our surroundings have the power to energize and uplift us ... or make us lethargic, depressed, or more susceptible to illnesses. In this chapter, we will discuss the basics of green design, talk about the components of a healthy environment, and provide some tips on becoming a savvier and more conscious consumer.

Green Design Basics

Green design, *eco design*, and *wellness design* are buzzwords you may have heard recently. If you're having trouble pinpointing what exactly they mean, that's okay! Green design encompasses a wide range of practices and philosophies and can refer to construction practices (e.g., recycling used materials), the materials and furnishings used in a building, a building's energy and water use, or even the overall setup of a space (e.g., choosing to include large south-facing windows to allow for more natural lighting). It is, perhaps, easiest to define green design by its overarching goal: to create a healthy environment using sustainable, responsibly sourced materials and eco-friendly construction and design practices.

On the one hand, green design is related to the health and well-being of a building's occupants. On the other hand, it is concerned with the health of the planet and the greater good. To help enhance healthy living for occupants, an eco-minded designer would, for example, choose toxin-free paints and flooring materials. To aid the planet and contribute to sustainability, that same designer might choose to incorporate recycled wood or use durable products that will last for decades.

Interior designers can choose to focus on any number of factors when it comes to improving a space's health and sustainability. When thinking about the occupants' health, it is important to use quality, allergen-free, nontoxic materials. It is also important to consider how the occupants interact with the space and how it can be optimized for mental, emotional, and physical health. For example, if an occupant works eight hours each day in a home office, it would be best for that person's well-being to have their desk situated near a window that lets in plenty of sunlight.

When considering sustainability, it is best to select quality, durable furnishings. Flimsy plastic or wooden products might be less expensive in the short term, but they will likely not hold up as well as quality materials and, therefore, have to be discarded much sooner.

Other sustainability best practices include purchasing responsibly sourced, locally produced, or recycled products or choosing upcycled products. Is the wood for a coffee table composed of endangered trees harvested from clear-cutting swaths of rain forest? Or is made from oak harvested fifty miles away?

Upcycled products are pre-owned items that have been repurposed or refurbished. While they are certainly a sustainable option, be aware that the previous owner's energy may still be lingering within the upcycled item—something Feng Shui consultants refer to as predecessor energy. If the lingering energy is positive and uplifting, that can have a beneficial effect, but if it is negative, that may cause problems or difficulties for you. In this case, it is best to work with a Feng Shui consultant who can make intentional corrections to clear the old energy and give you and the pre-owned object a fresh start.

Another sustainability consideration has to do with the eventual disposal of a product. Can it be easily recycled or repurposed? Or is it doomed to end up in a landfill?

Why Choose Green Design?

As an interior designer, a mother, and a responsible citizen, I have made it my professional goal to embrace green design. That's why I decided to become a green accredited professional. This professional certification is granted by the Sustainable Furnishings Council, an organization dedicated to promoting eco-friendly practices in the home furnishings industry. As a green accredited professional, I endeavor to minimize carbon emissions, avoid unrecyclable or toxic materials, stem the flow of waste stream pollutants, and use materials from sustainable sources whenever possible. This discipline is broad and ever growing, which means I am constantly learning about different aspects of green design.

Did you know that nearly 40 percent of greenhouse gas emissions (which contribute to global warming) are caused by buildings?[10] That is a *staggering* figure, and it is up to contractors, builders, interior designers, *and* consumers to be change-makers when it comes to green design. Climate change is no longer an abstract threat or a remote possibility; it is a very real danger that has manifested itself in record-high temperatures, melting sea ice, and increasingly erratic weather phenomenon (from droughts to intense wildfires to record-setting hurricane seasons). All the carbon and pollutants that we've released into the atmosphere are beginning to take their toll, and it is up to us to make responsible choices for our children and for generations to come.

How do buildings compose 40 percent of greenhouse gas emissions? The link between buildings and emissions is not as obvious as vehicles, which spew pollutants out of their tailpipes. Rather, buildings can cause an environmental burden because they are so multifaceted. Not only do they consume plenty of energy (through electric lights, air conditioning units, water heaters, etc.), but they are also made of many different components. Think about a simple front door. The metal or wood composing the door has to be mined or harvested. The glass must be manufactured. The paint must be made. The metal hardware needs to be mined and then manufactured. All these parts must come together in a factory, be assembled, and then

---

10. "Buildings & Built Infrastructure."

be shipped to a warehouse or home improvement store. Then, a vehicle hauls the door to your home. And that's just a door! Think about all the infrastructure and furnishings that compose a building—all the copper or PVC pipes, the flooring, cabinetry, bathtubs, ceiling fans, electric wiring, gutters, and much, much more. Each component has to be harvested or mined *somewhere*, and each component needs to be manufactured and shipped. And on top of that, a home consumes energy. It uses electricity and gobbles either natural gas or propane.

The simple truth is that buildings are complicated. They consist of many different resources and are often operated by fossil fuels (nonrenewable resources, such as natural gas, oil, and coal). However, each step of the way we have the opportunity to make healthy, eco-conscious choices. And our choices are powerful. We can encourage timber companies to practice ethical harvesting. We can make toxin-free materials the norm rather than the exception. We can reduce landfill waste and cut down on electricity use. Our collective choices can carve out a better future *while* we're creating a healthier, nourishing home environment.

Even you, as an individual consumer, can make an immediate impact. How? Start by improving the health of your home environment.

Creating a Healthy Environment

You don't have to be a green designer to make a positive impact on your living space. There are many small steps you can take to create a healthier home or a more livable workspace. Your design choices can influence your productivity, energy, and overall health. I have often witnessed how even small changes in a home can improve the occupants' well-being and ability to thrive.

Years ago, when I sensed my marriage was in trouble, I began to actively build my business to increase my financial stability. With that goal in mind, I leased a two-story Victorian home, which housed my office and, eventually, served as a living space while I went through my divorce.

The historic home was beautiful, but it was falling into disrepair and had been chronically neglected by past occupants. Additionally, the space felt cluttered, and the air seemed musty. The exterior wall was dotted with small holes where rodents could potentially crawl in. In short, the space was plagued with bad energy.

This bad energy was apparent when you stepped inside the building, and it had a noticeable effect on past occupants since many stayed in the space for only a few months. However, I was determined to improve the environment using the principles of Feng Shui as well as green design elements.

With the owner's permission, I set about remodeling or adjusting parts of the building. I identified potentially harmful elements in the space and went about fixing them. I also added personal touches, such as beautiful window treatments and a stylish showroom for my business. I even hired a dowser who used metal dowsing rods to locate energy fields, pinpoint areas of negative energy, and rebalance the energy. All these steps were a labor of love for me as well as a way to create a wholly positive space while my personal life was taking a difficult turn.

Not long after making these changes, the atmosphere of the old Victorian building completely changed. The energy seemed brighter and more vibrant, and the environmental health noticeably improved. All the changes I had made helped ground the space and invited positivity and vibrancy, which, in turn, propelled my business and allowed me to be more successful and prosperous.

I eventually found other living accommodations and a new office space, but that ancient Victorian house served me well until the day I moved out. The individual who leased the space after me was a responsible long-term tenant whom my landlord knew and trusted—further evidence that my revamp of the house had brought a newfound stability to the space.

The Components of a Healthy Environment

When thinking about the health of an indoor environment, there are many factors to consider. One important factor is air. Air is integral to our health and well-being. Have you ever stepped into a room that was so musty you had an instant reaction to it? Or have you been in a place with zero airflow? In the 1970s and beyond, it became very common for buildings to be sealed tight with little air exchange. This building design choice led to a condition known as "sick building syndrome," in which interior toxins became trapped in the home and often made their way into the occupants' bodies.

Our lungs are not meant to breathe contaminated or stagnant air, and it's no coincidence that more and more people are developing asthma or chronic respiratory issues every year. Today, one out of every thirteen Americans—about twenty-five *million* people—has asthma.[11] To improve air quality in a room, focus on reducing dust, purchase a quality air purifier, eliminate any dampness or mold, and make sure there is ample air exchange. You might also consider hiring an air quality professional to inspect your home (search for an indoor air quality [IAQ] specialist online to find a list of professionals in your area).

Another factor that can undermine the health of an environment are toxins. Unfortunately, toxins can be found in many common household products and materials. Even though the national Environmental Protection Agency (EPA) does ban some of these harmful products (lead pipes, for example, and asbestos), regulations are often slow to catch up with science (and common knowledge!) or are not very stringent. For example, the

---

11. Goff, "Asthma Facts and Figures."

EPA regulates VOCs in *some* products but not others. VOCs, or volatile organic compounds, are harmful chemicals that can be found in paints, dry cleaning products, refrigerants, and more. These chemicals can cause adverse health symptoms ranging from headaches to allergic reactions to hormonal disruption.

You might also find harmful toxins in the glue that was used for your flooring, in the asbestos integrated into many vinyl tiles or older walls or ceilings, or in the formaldehyde found in some pressed wood products or synthetic fabrics. Even your mattress could be a haven for toxic materials. Since 2007 mattresses have been required to be flame resistant, and many mattress companies have opted to use potent chemicals to get the job done. These chemicals have potentially disastrous side effects, including skin irritation, lung damage, immune system suppression, endocrine and thyroid disruption, and cancer. And those are just some of the known side effects. Fortunately, consumers are speaking out against the use of flame-retardant chemicals in mattresses and several mattress companies are now using chemical-free covers or nontoxic materials, such as naturally flame-retardant wool or plant-based memory foam.

In addition to eliminating toxins, it's also important to avoid materials that may cause allergic reactions. Some people may be allergic to synthetic fabrics, for example, or certain dyes or glues, and many people are allergic to dust, which can easily collect in dense cushions. If you are allergic to dust or dander, consider covering your pillows and mattress with allergen-proof cases or finding an eco-friendly cleaning service for your upholstery (search online for "green cleaning" or "eco-friendly cleaning" to get started).

If you'd like to improve the health of your indoor environment, do your research and search for products that are both toxin/allergen-free and environmentally friendly. Here are a few ideas:

+ Avoid veneers. These wooden tops can be laden with harmful chemicals.
+ Look for chemical-free mattresses. Latex from the rapidly renewable rubber tree makes an excellent nontoxic mattress or cushion fill.
+ Avoid polyurethane foam fill in furniture. Wool, kapok, and down are better alternatives, *and* they are biodegradable. Wool is also a natural flame retardant.
+ Avoid vinyl flooring or harmful wood glues. Vinyl can release toxic chemicals that can lead to serious diseases, such as cancer, or cause birth defects. Alternate flooring choices include bamboo, cork, solid wood, or phthalates-free vinyl flooring.
+ Seek rugs and carpeting that do not use synthetic fibers or backing. The Healthy Building Network recently identified forty-four toxic chemicals

found in conventional carpeting.[12] Instead, look
for alternatives that incorporate materials such as
jute, wool, organic cotton, or silk.

EMFs in Your Environment

An often overlooked health risk associated with interior
spaces are EMFs, or electromagnetic fields. Though the earth
produces natural electromagnetic fields, human activity has
greatly increased their presence over the past century. EMFs
are synonymous with nonionizing radiation. They can be tol-
erated by most healthy people in low amounts, but they can
potentially cause harm when the strength of the fields rises,
regardless of whether the EMFs have lower frequencies with
longer wavelengths, such as magnetic and electric fields from
household wiring, or higher frequencies with shorter wavelengths, such as those from wireless transmitters. Common
household sources of EMFs are microwaves, heat lamps, electric lights, cell phones, and wireless internet.

Though several high-profile experts assert that nonionizing EMFs are mostly harmless, other sources dispute that
claim. In my own research, I have found several studies that
demonstrate the potential harmful effects of EMFs, which
can include poor sleep, depression, reduced immune function, and certain types of cancer. Naturally, I err on the side of

---

12. Vallette, Stamm, and Lent, "Eliminating Toxics in Carpet: Lessons for
the Future of Recycling."

caution and recommend reducing EMFs in the home wherever possible.

Remember the old Victorian house I remodeled? When I was in the midst of overhauling the building, I decided it would be prudent to call upon a building biologist to measure the EMFs in the building and pinpoint any potential trouble spots. The discipline of building biology, or *baubiologie*, was founded in Germany with the intention of treating the home as an extension of ourselves. The building is viewed almost like a living organism whose health must be examined and enhanced whenever possible. A building biologist looks at a building from a holistic standpoint and takes into consideration the air quality, water (usage and purity), out-gassing from building materials, overall building design, environmental sustainability, and electric, magnetic, and radio frequency fields.

Building biologists can specialize in specific areas, and I decided to call upon an electromagnetic radiation specialist (EMRS) named Oram Miller to assist with the Victorian house. Oram is also a certified building biology environmental consultant (BBEC). He received his certifications from the Building Biology Institute in Santa Fe, New Mexico. He is a respected expert in the field and has given numerous radio and podcast interviews and delivered several lectures. He currently teaches electromagnetic radiation courses as an adjunct faculty for the Building Biology Institute. Today, he lives and works in the Los Angeles area, helping clients in Southern California and around the country.[13]

Oram was a true professional and gave the building a thorough sweep with his many meters, including a gauss meter, a device that measures electrical currents in milligauss (mG), and a radio frequency meter, which measures Wi-Fi and cellular frequencies. As Oram went through the house, he identified several areas that surpassed recommended EMF levels according to his profession. One particularly potent area was a snarl of electrical and cable/telephone wires right outside my bedroom window. This was especially troubling since bedrooms are supposed to be an area of rest and rejuvenation, and electric field EMFs from nonmetallic, plastic-jacketed Romex circuits in bedroom walls and floors can directly interfere with the depth and quality of our natural sleep cycles.

Oram's readings made me aware of potential problems in the home, and he gave me the information I needed to make a few important changes. If you're worried about EMFs in your home, you can purchase your own EMF meters or, better yet, hire an EMF expert like Oram to assist you. Even if you do not fully eliminate EMF sources in your home, you can still take preventative measures, such as moving certain electronic devices away from sitting areas or adjusting electrical cords that you plug in near where you sit. Oram's website, www .createhealthyhomes.com, has many articles in the education

---

13. "Bio for Oram Miller."

section that will guide you on how to identify and reduce EMFs in your home along with having a building biologist or other EMF expert assess where you live and work.

Other preventative steps include:

+ Never use a laptop on your lap or abdomen.
+ Convert from Wi-Fi to hardwired (ethernet) connections for internet access; turn off Wi-Fi and Bluetooth on your computer.
+ Do not run electrical cords beneath your bed, chairs, or tables.
+ Turn off your phone's Bluetooth function unless you are using it (or, better yet, use a corded landline telephone at home).
+ Keep your sleeping area as EMF-free as possible, which includes avoiding electric clocks and electric blankets, and have your bedroom checked by a building biologist for electric fields.

Becoming a Smart Consumer

With so much conflicting information and countless resources available, it can be difficult to be a smart, savvy consumer. Where do you begin? How is it possible to buy furnishings or materials that are nontoxic *and* made from responsibly sourced materials *and* affordable? Fortunately, with an increasing number of consumers demanding change, it's getting easier to find quality, ethical goods at a reasonable price point. A quick internet search should lead you to a number of sustainable goods, from bamboo flooring to recycled wood countertops. Even so, it's a good idea to be on the lookout for companies and products that *claim* to be sustainable but have no proof to back up that claim.

At times, consumers' hearts are in the right place, but they fear that "going green" will be too expensive. While that can be true in some circumstances, it certainly isn't always the case, especially when you consider the long-term return on your investment. For instance, a low-flow toilet, an energy-saving refrigerator, or a high-efficiency furnace can actually be cheaper in the long run when you take energy savings into account. Additionally, eco-friendly furnishings and appliances are getting increasingly common, which also helps to drive down the price.

If you're looking to purchase products from responsible companies, one way to find them is to look for labels of approval from regulatory programs. Each of these programs has a set of standards that a company must follow in order to earn their label. Examples include:

> **Various sustainable forestry programs** such as Programme for the Endorsement of Forest Certification (PEFC), Sustainable Forestry Initiative (SFI), and Forest Stewardship Council (FSC).
>
> **Fair trade programs** that promote practices such as fair worker wages, the enforcement of labor laws,

and environmental stewardship. These organizations include Fairtrade International, Fair Trade USA, and the World Fair Trade Organization (WFTO).

Programs that focus on cutting pollution or carbon, including CarbonCare and Climate Neutral Product Certification.

Other eco certification programs, including Eco3Home (certifies sustainable furnishings), GreenCircle (verifies sustainability of products and manufacturing operations; recommended by the EPA), SCS (certifies sustainable carpeting), and NSF (focused on commercial fabrics).

Another approach to becoming an eco-minded consumer is to buy local products from trusted sources. If, for instance, someone in your community weaves baskets or builds dining room tables from locally sourced or recycled wood, why not give them your business? It may not be as expensive as you think to patronize a local artisan since you'll be cutting out all the middlemen (the distributors, warehousers, and big box stores). If you're not sure where to look, check out local farmer's markets or attend an artisan fair.

Your Turn

If you'd like to get started on improving the health and sustainability of your space, it's a good idea to begin with the items that may be the most problematic:

1. **Eliminate potential sources of toxins.**

    Start your green design journey in one room and begin to identify potential sources of toxins. Are there any synthetic materials present in the room? What is your rug or carpeting made of, and does it have a traditional rubber backing? What materials are used in your sofa cushions, chairs, and pillows? Do you potentially have asbestos in your ceiling or walls? Vinyl flooring? Walls painted with old paint? All these areas are potential havens for toxins.

    When removing sources of toxins, exercise caution! Some materials are fine to handle on your own, but others, such as asbestos, require the assistance of a qualified professional for removal and disposal.

2. **Identify sources of EMFs.**

    The first step in protecting yourself from the potential harm of radiation is to understand the main sources of EMFs in your home. Either purchase a gauss meter or hire an EMF expert to map your home and identify the areas where radiation is especially strong. After that, you can go about eliminating some of these electrical sources (do you really need a nightlight in your bedroom?), shifting some of them (moving your router farther away from your desk, for instance), or avoiding them when they are running (such as stepping away from your microwave when it is operating). Remember: It's a good idea to eliminate as many sources of radiation as possible from your bedroom to create a restful environment.

3. **Recycle/Upcycle**

   If you're planning to get rid of certain items in your home, don't just throw them in the trash! Many items can be recycled, although you may not be able to simply toss them into your recycling bin. Specialized recycling facilities may take items such as laminate flooring, old paint, construction debris (including wood waste and plastics), mattresses, electronics, copper wiring, or stone countertops. Search online for "specialized recycling" in your area to find recycling facilities near you. Additionally your energy provider may have a program in place for recycling old appliances, such as refrigerators or washing machines.

If you can't recycle certain items, consider upcycling or donating them. Repurpose old asphalt shingles by using them to roof a playhouse or doghouse. Upcycle cracked tiles for a mosaic-style garden path. If you are getting rid of light fixtures, faucets, or vintage furnishings (like a clawfoot bathtub), consider donating them or posting about them on social media. You never know what others might be seeking.

Though no one expects you to be a *perfect* consumer, we can all try a little harder when it comes to sustainability and ethical choices. Do your best to educate yourself, understand the options that are available to you, and make your interior design decisions only after you've done your due diligence. If you need further guidance, consult a green accredited professional designer to help you with your décor decisions.

Chapter 10
Changing Life, Changing Space

I t is said that the same river will never pass by the same spot twice. That is because a river is constantly in motion, ever changing. It picks up nutrients and deposits them. It carves new tracks through sediment and rock. It swells during times of rain and diminishes during droughts.

Like a river, people also have a tendency to shift and change with seasons and circumstances. We are influenced by new people and experiences. We grow as we acquire knowledge, skills, and beliefs. Sometimes, we change in profound ways, and sometimes, the changes are gradual and subtle.

Change is normal and natural—an essential part of life. Year by year, we become different versions of ourselves as we age, develop new friendships and relationships (or redefine old ones), and modify our aspirations. And yet, our homes, workplaces, and other personal spaces do not always reflect the people we've become or aspire to become.

When that happens, you might feel a sense of "wrongness" in certain spaces, feeling like a hermit crab that's outgrown its shell. If you feel that way about an area of your home or workplace, I encourage you to listen to your intuition. If your space no longer mirrors your life circumstances, it may be time for a design change, Feng Shui adjustments, or even a remodel.

I have worked with many people who have decided to overhaul their living or workspace because they experienced a major life alteration. Some of these individuals had already designed their space using Feng Shui principles, but after a time, their lives had changed, and they needed to refresh their space. A significant change might occur when two people combine households, when a couple welcomes their first child, or when a person's career goals change significantly. Not long ago, I worked with a couple whose household dynamics changed after their children grew up and moved away from their family home.

After the Kanes became empty nesters, their house began to feel … *off*. Their adult children's bedrooms sat vacant much of the time, and the rooms were essentially frozen in time, filled with relics of childhood. Once their adult children began starting careers and families of their own, the Kanes knew it was time to modify these areas so they were comfortable and inviting for their children and their spouses. They wanted to convey that their kids were welcome to stay in the family home at any time.

With that goal in mind, the Kanes took on the attitude of: "If you build it, they will come." They resolved to intentionally create a space that would appeal to their children and entice them to stay overnight whenever they were in the area.

Working closely together, the Kanes and I made Feng Shui–centric design choices that revolved around creating a tranquil and welcoming atmosphere. We removed clutter and intentionally selected colors and artwork that conveyed a sense of calm and were easy on the eye. To create a couple's haven, we replaced the old bunk beds with a queen-sized bed (king-sized beds have a tendency to create distance between couples) and chose to *not* place a TV in the room, which can lead to poor sleep and health issues (see chapter 9's discussion on EMFs in the bedroom).

We also incorporated specific symbols in the bedroom that related to both tranquility and a bright, promising future. Behind the bed, we installed a solid headboard to facilitate a sense of support and the feeling of stability. Conversely, we did *not* hang shelves over the bed since that placement can create unease or instability (which no one wants in a bedroom!). The artwork we selected was rich with symbolism. One painting showed a forest path with light trickling through the branches, which conveys growth and a positive path ahead. Two other paintings, hung side by side over the bed, displayed contemporary-looking wildflowers. Flowers are closely related to fire energy and wood energy—two of the five elements. Their symbolic fire energy can nurture enthusiasm and passion, and their wood energy encourages growth.

Though the room incorporated a touch of nostalgia (we displayed some of the kids' trophies on a shelving unit across from the bed), it was primarily a practical space meant to cater to its guests. We included a charging station for smartphones, a long bench where guests could sit and remove their shoes, and an end table with an attached lamp. An attached bathroom allowed for privacy and convenience, and a walk-in closet provided plenty of space for guests to hang their clothing or temporarily store personal items.

Once completed, the Kanes' new guest room became an inviting and cozy space to welcome back their six children and their spouses. It reflected the Kanes' current reality and helped them embrace life as empty nesters rather than resist it.

Facing Change

It is not always easy to cope with major life changes. Sometimes, we yearn for things to remain the same ("I wish my children would remain small forever." "If only my marriage were as healthy and exciting as it once was." "I wish my friend wasn't moving away."). But regrets and wishes are not useful when it comes to change. Life marches forward, whether we want it to or not, and the healthiest way to deal with change is to face it.

One effective way to confront change is to spend time in meaningful reflection. Set aside quiet time for yourself to contemplate your life's circumstances and ponder your future. There is no "right way" to do this, and your reflection time might look quite different from someone else's. You might, for example, choose to meditate in the morning while practicing gentle yoga. Or you might choose to go on a morning stroll.

Or you could write your thoughts in a reflection journal each morning or evening. The energy tools I outlined in chapter 3 (especially journaling and practicing breathing techniques) are great ways to engage in self-reflection.

As you begin practicing self-reflection, try different methods and stick with whatever works for you—whatever feels comfortable. The important thing is not the method; it's what you gain from your reflection. Ultimately your goal is to develop a better understanding of yourself and your present circumstances. To stay in tune with yourself, it's a good idea to engage in self-reflection on a regular basis. Even setting aside ten minutes each day can be helpful. Think of this time as your chance to "check in" with yourself and see how you're doing.

During these check-ins, it's a good idea to occasionally contemplate your space and surroundings and consider whether or not they still serve their intended purposes. Does your bedroom, for instance, reflect the type of energy you'd like to attract to that space? Does your office reflect your aspirations? Do you avoid certain parts of your home because the energy feels "off"? Is your living space helping to cultivate your goals and dreams? If you're having difficulty pinpointing your feelings about certain spaces, refer to the emotional scale chart in chapter 5.

When thinking about changing your space to match your life's circumstances, you might begin to feel daunted or overwhelmed. I challenge you to reframe your thinking. Instead of fearing change, think of it as an opportunity—a closed door waiting to be opened. Begin to open yourself to possibilities and welcome the potential for personal development and growth.

You might also try practicing visualization in which you picture yourself in the future—*after* you've adjusted or remodeled your space. What blessings have entered your life because of the change you've facilitated? What opportunities have presented themselves? How has your outlook on life changed? Visualization is a powerful tool used by successful entrepreneurs, professional athletes, and TV personalities alike. It has become wildly popular in recent years because it works! Imagining your future successes can help you determine the best path to take to achieve them.

Keep in mind, changing your space doesn't have to be intimidating. It can be undertaken gradually—at a pace that matches your comfort level. Besides, you do not have to embark on this journey alone. Enlisting the help of a Feng Shui interior designer can help you get started, and they can provide the support you need to overhaul your home or workplace.

Ultimately, revamping your space should be enjoyable. I like to encourage people to not take their home redesigns so seriously and to find joy in remodeling or redecorating. Remember my concept of the Fun Shui Way? Take that message to heart, have fun, and let your unique self shine.

Embracing change and deciding to redo your space are vital steps toward carving out a better future for yourself. Your engines are started, and you're ready to take off. But not so fast! Before you dive headlong into a home or office revamp, it is important to consider the space and how to adjust it to your needs. Let's talk about how to do that.

Remodeling/Adjusting Your Space

When considering how to remodel or adjust your space, it's helpful to think about your most important or urgent goals. What changes would you like to invite into your life in the near future? What old habits or harmful relationships would you like to reject? What are your professional goals? (If you need a refresher on goal setting, refer to chapter 2.)

By keeping your goals at the top of your mind, you'll be better able to approach your space with a forward-thinking lens. If, for example, your goal is to attract a new partner, it's a good idea to examine your bedroom and ponder whether or not the space is inviting. Are the paint colors suited to the energy you would like to foster? Is the bed sized correctly? Are there two nightstands (one on each side of the bed) and two lamps? Is there extra space in your closet for additional clothes, or is it packed to the gills?

When you have a clear idea of your goals, it can be easier to look around your space and identify what might be holding you back. Of course, some goals may require less obvious changes or adjustments. In those cases, it is useful to refer to Feng Shui handbooks or get in touch with an expert consultant who can pinpoint areas that can be improved and recommend personalized changes.

Specific rooms can benefit from specific adjustments or design choices. I will address some room recommendations later in this section, but first I'd like to reiterate that certain Feng Shui basics can improve the energy of *any* room. These basics include decluttering (are there too many objects crowding the floors or walls?), having a clear intention for the space, improving the energy flow (and clearing out negative energy), and making sure the room is well balanced. Much of this advice boils down to one concept: simplicity.

The most comfortable, classic rooms are often those that adhere to simple design concepts and only include a few key accents, such as artwork, an elemental symbol or two (a stone or water feature, for example), an eye-catching coffee table, or a pop of color. One benefit of keeping designs simple is that it is easy to make adjustments to a room if you'd like to alter its energy or shift your intentions for the space. Additionally, by keeping designs simple, you can invest in a few high-quality pieces (rather than several mediocre ones), which can elevate the look and feel of the room *and* can also be eco-friendly (if you're using sustainable materials that will last a long time).

These basic Feng Shui practices can be applied to any room, but specific rooms are also associated with specific recommendations. I am going to discuss several rooms within the home and deliver a few useful pieces of advice that can help you overhaul or revitalize your space.

Keep in mind, these recommendations only scratch the surface of what is possible in your home, and they should be used in conjunction with other Feng Shui best practices.

Bedrooms

When I started in the interior design business, people would ask which area they should fix or decorate first to improve their homes. My mentor's answer was to start with the entryway because that is the first area everyone sees when entering your home.

After attending Feng Shui school, I learned that one's bedroom is actually a more powerful starting point for home redesign; however, my mentor was not entirely incorrect. The entryway and, by extension, the front door, is an essential component of home design. The front door is considered the mouth of chi. It is a main channel for letting energy into the home. By painting your front door a bold color—something that contrasts with the color of the home's siding—you invite positive energy to enter the home. It is also a good idea to regularly use your front door to help energy flow inside. If you tend to use a different door to enter your home, I suggest walking through the front door at least once per week. Honor your front door by framing it nicely, painting it a pleasant color or surrounding it with columns, decorative vases, or statues. By making your front door stand out, you are guiding positive, vibrant energy into your home.

Despite the importance of the front door and entryway, I encourage you to begin your redesign work in the main bedroom. This space is powerful because it is where we rest and restore ourselves; it provides us with much-needed energy to rise and face the day's challenges. Working on the main bedroom first is an act of self-care, and it, in turn, will raise your vibration and energy level to continue with other areas of your home and life. Once you're well rested and feeling good, you can move on to refining and decorating other rooms in your home.

We spend about a third of our lives in the bedroom. It is a place of rest, rejuvenation, and romance. Because we spend so much time in this deeply personal space, it can have a profound effect on our lives. Therefore, it is of utmost importance to invite positive, harmonious energy into the bedroom and to foster a sense of tranquility.

Creating a calm, harmonious bedroom starts with a wall color you love that feels relaxing to you. Some of my favorite wall colors for bedrooms are soft teals, greens, and neutral tones, such as a soft taupe. Reds and yellows are more energetic and can keep you up at night, so it's best to have toned-down colors if you are sensitive to brighter colors. You might choose to add bolder colors in smaller amounts in the artwork or decorative accessories. Most importantly, it is crucial to love the color you choose for your walls.

How does your bedroom nurture you? Is it helping you find peace amidst the chaos of the outside world? The following is a list of elements and ideas to create a more luxurious and relaxing bedroom:

- Add soft window treatments, such as draperies, drapery panels, roman shades, or valances over blinds, that control the light.
- Add dimmer switches to the lighting so you can adjust for reading, relaxing, or romance. LED lights now come in an array of colors and have wide-ranging dimmable features. Smart lights can be controlled by a phone app or voice commands.
- Choose bed sheets that are soft and luxurious. Select colors that relax and appeal to you.
- Having a solid headboard will help you feel more supported.
- If you are part of a couple or would like to attract a partner, it is best to have two nightstands.
- Place the bed so you can see the door but not so it is directly aligned with it (command position).
- Move desks or exercise equipment elsewhere. Such items create too much energy for a space to be relaxing. Having a desk in your bedroom will subconsciously remind you of work, and exercise equipment is too stimulating to induce rest.

+ Minimize electronics (including electric blankets) and avoid installing a TV in the bedroom. These items are the antithesis of tranquility and can also emit harmful EMFs (see chapter 9). If a TV must go in the bedroom, keep it concealed in an armoire or cover it at night with an attractive-looking blanket.
+ Use mirrors with caution. They can create overly active energy in the bedroom and impede sleep. If you have a visible mirror, drape a blanket or piece of cloth over it at night.
+ Bring in sensual or serene artwork.
+ Avoid placing your bed beneath low beams or shelving, and do not store items under the bed. These factors can subconsciously cause stress and disquiet.

Following these guidelines doesn't restrict you to designing an unappealing space. Any style can be adapted, whether it's casual or elegant. It's all about finding a pleasing level of comfort. Adding adequate storage and putting electronic equipment behind doors contributes to creating a peaceful, uncluttered environment. As I like to say: "A place for everything and everything in its well-designed place."

Kitchen

According to Feng Shui tradition, the kitchen is the heart of the home since we spend so much time and convene there. It represents health, wealth, and nourishment. It is an active area that facilitates family gatherings and food preparation. Kitchens are usually associated with the fire element, which is directly linked to the stove, oven, and cooking in general.

+ The best placement (typically) for a kitchen is at the back of the home. Kitchens located toward the front have an immediate tug on the occupants when they walk through the door, which can cause eating or digestive disorders. Kitchens located in the home's center can cause an overabundance of fire energy. Since a home's center is representative of health, too much fire energy can feel like an attack and can usher in bad energy.

+ Knives should not be displayed in plain view or kept on the countertop but instead should be concealed in a drawer organizer insert.

+ Keep horizontal surfaces free of clutter.

+ The stove symbolizes your resources and career. Its energy is most effective when placed in the command position, which allows whoever is using the stove to see the entryway (and whoever is coming or going). A kitchen island is an excellent location for a stove, but if that is not a possibility, a mirror can be placed above the stove as an adjustment to provide a view of whoever enters the room. I have placed mirrors in this manner in three of my homes, and they have proven to be quite tolerant of heat and easy to clean.

Dining Room

The dining room is a place for relaxation and enjoyment. It can create harmony in the home, strengthen family bonds, and foster joy.

+ Comfort and security are important in a dining room. If possible, avoid seating that places the occupants' backs to the windows or door as this can create a sense of vulnerability.
+ Adding mirrors to a dining room increases prosperity by doubling the abundance of what you have on your table.
+ To aid in digestion, select artwork that is calming.
+ Choose a round or oval table, if possible, because its energy is less confrontational than a rectangular table and more relaxing. If you do happen to have a rectangular table, counteract its effect by placing an oval throw rug beneath it.
+ To avoid getting in a rut, sit in every seat at the dining room table. This helps you see your home

from different angles and view what your guests
or family members see.

Family/Living Room

A family room or living room is a center for cheer and camara-
derie. It is typically a central social space and is often associated
with abundance, health, and happiness. Unlike a bedroom or
a dining room, a family room can be a place to foster an energetic, bright atmosphere.

Indestructibility can be an important feature of living areas, depending on the age of the occupants. Anyone with a
young child should be (and probably already is) mindful of objects that break easily or could scrape or cut the child. If older
adults live in the space, the design should also focus on safety
and comfort (e.g., utilizing floors that are not slippery or selecting furniture that is not too low to the ground) in addition
to indestructibility. For occupants of any age, it's a good idea to
not use too many fragile or easily stained materials in a living
area. Choose fabrics that are easy to clean and can camouflage
minor stains.

Here are a few more family room tips:

+ Make sure the room is equipped with adequate
  storage to keep it clutter free. It is important to
  keep family rooms clear to create good energy
  flow and promote vitality and health.
+ Conceal electronics behind closed doors.

+ Select colors and artwork that are bright, cheerful, and evoke joy.
+ Choose furniture that is tasteful but also casual and inviting for the room's occupants to enjoy.
+ Select flooring and furniture that are both comfortable and as indestructible as possible.

Bathroom

The bathroom's primary function is to cleanse our body inside and out. Decorate your bathroom beautifully and keep it clutter free. Paint bathrooms any color you'd like as long as it flows with the rest of your structure. Vibrant, deep colors are just as wonderful as light, airy ones, depending on the look you want. If you choose darker colors, add lighting that is adequate for the environment. Dimmer switches will give you the option to brighten or dim the area for a spa-like feel.

Bathrooms can be tricky areas in the home. From a Feng Shui perspective, plumbing is a potential threat to energy circulation, or chi. Open toilet lids and drains can potentially deplete energy, while the overwhelming presence of water can create an elemental imbalance. However, there are several steps you can take to cultivate a clean, pleasant environment and channel the power of water to promote wealth, personal growth, and renewal.

+ To avoid energy drains, keep your bathroom door closed, cover the drains, and keep your toilet lid down. Always repair leaking faucets immediately.

+ If possible, install the toilet so it is not visible from the door.

+ Avoid placing mirrors that reflect the toilet as this can double the draining effect.

+ Focus on making your bathroom beautiful and inviting. Since wood absorbs water, it can be a good idea to include representations of the wood element in your bathroom if you have an overabundance of water energy. You might also try incorporating the earth element as well to channel or contain water energy.

+ Place a plant or unpopped popcorn on the back of your toilet to elevate the energy of the room. A plant signifies upward growth and counteracts the draining energy of the toilet. Similarly, un-popped popcorn has "lifting" energy, which will pull the energy of the space upward and offset draining influences.

+ Scrub your bathroom often, keep it clean, and incorporate pleasant fragrances whenever possible.

Design for Utilitarian Spaces

No area of the home should be neglected, including garages, attics, basements, and mudrooms. Beautify these spaces with epoxy floors, painted walls, fun industrial-styled lighting, and attractive cabinets. If any furniture, shelving, or accessories are broken, they can subconsciously promote anxiety or evoke negative emotions. Either eliminate or repair broken items.

If you're using these areas for storage, make sure you only store items you love and use. Keep those items well organized and labeled so you always know where to find them.

I encourage you to put artwork on the walls in these areas, too. Think about how you will feel when you pull into the garage and view an inspiring piece of artwork. This can influence your mood when you walk through the door and into your home, setting the tone for your relationship with yourself, family, friends, and even your pets.

One commonly neglected space is the laundry room or mudroom. These are usually considered utilitarian spaces, but that doesn't mean they have to look the part! Because they're the place where families likely enter the home (or, at the very least, use frequently), they must be functional, organized, and attractive. The design of these areas should not only look good but also feel good.

Blend beauty and purpose in your laundry and mudroom design with these tips:

+ **Stray from the norm.** Instead of an afterthought, make your laundry/mudroom atypical with upgraded materials, fun colors, uplifting artwork, and unique accent pieces that lift your spirits.

+ **Make it cohesive.** Blend the look and feel with the rest of the home to ensure a seamless transition from room to room, coordinating the overall aesthetics.

+ **Build it in.** Be thoughtful about what you want to store and where and strive for convenience. Build a little extra space into your design to use for items such as sporting goods, seasonal items, hobby/crafting tools, and more. Use cabinets with pullout drawers and bins to hide things out of sight and create a streamlined look.

Most importantly, make your laundry/mudroom a space you enjoy when you come home.

Feng Shui Tools

Adjusting or remodeling individual rooms can be a powerful way to reclaim your space and pave the way to a better future. Sometimes, however, minor adjustments are all that is needed to uplift a space or create a better energy flow. I've already mentioned decluttering, rebalancing a room, and choosing simplicity as methods for improving energy, but there are several more tactics you can try. One approach you might take for revitalizing your space is using certain tools to make specific energetic changes.

Feng Shui Tools

LIGHT & LIGHT-REFRACTING OBJECTS

Mirrors:

- Guide and direct the flow of chi
- Draw in auspicious chi
- Expand an area or reflect an area
- Move an area totally
- Allow chi to penetrate closed spaces
- Counter a negative influence by turning it upside down

Crystals:

- Adjust direction of chi
- Slow down chi in long hallways
- Fill out a missing piece in the Bagua
- Enhance the general health of the individual or business if placed in the exact center of the space
- Increase visualization and clarity around an issue

Lights:

- Lift rooms with low ceilings or beams
- Fill out a missing piece of the Bagua
- Enhance a dark corner or section of the Bagua

HEAVY OBJECTS

Stones & Statues:

- Bring balance and stability
- Bring wholeness to a missing piece of the Bagua
- Elicit strength and power when needed

SOUND-MAKING OBJECTS

Chimes & Bells:
- Alert or awaken the mind
- Call out for an answer
- Call out for clarity
- Lift the energy of the chi
- Bring good luck

Bamboo Flutes:
- Provide strength and support
- Bring peace into your life
- Guard and protect

WATER OBJECTS

Fountains & Aquariums:
- Symbolize wealth and prosperity
- Fill out a missing piece of the Bagua

LIVING OBJECTS

Plants & Flowers:
- Bring growth and potential
- Bring good luck

When you're going through a life change (whether major or minor), it can be beneficial to tap into the power of Feng Shui tools and objects to ease you through the transition. Some of these tools have been used for millennia to improve the energy in a space or redirect the chi. The following is a list of some tools and techniques to try. Keep in mind that this is not an exhaustive list, and many more tools exist that can help you make necessary adjustments.

Light-Refracting Objects

Mirrors are one of the more common Feng Shui tools; they are highly effective and have a variety of uses. They can guide or direct the flow of chi, draw in auspicious chi, or allow chi to penetrate closed spaces. If an area of the Bagua is missing, a mirror could be used to create that space. Mirrors can also counter harmful influences by acting as a buffer that distorts negative energy. Since mirrors are so powerful, they should be used with caution to avoid amplifying negative energy or over-energizing a space that is meant to be tranquil.

Crystals are another type of light-refracting object. Like mirrors, they can also be used to adjust the direction of chi or to slow its flow in long hallways. If placed in the precise center of a space, crystals can enhance the overall health of the occupants of a home or business. Many Feng Shui consultants use crystals to amplify visualization or improve clarity around an issue.

Lights are not exactly "light refracting" but are instead a source of illumination. As such, they have the power to uplift the energy in a room by lighting a dark corner or section of the Bagua. Balance your space with a mix of overhead lights and lamps and consider adding accent lighting to draw attention to certain features or influence the mood of the room. Lights can also provide "lift" to rooms with low ceilings or beams. Choose lights that are not too glaring or artificial but instead mimic natural outdoor lighting.

Heavy Objects

When your space is in need of grounding, heavy objects can facilitate this type of energy. These objects include stones and statues, and they can be used in both indoor and outdoor spaces. Heavy objects can provide stability and balance in many areas of the Bagua, including knowledge, health, and relationships. They can also bring wholeness to a missing piece of the Bagua. It is a good idea to intentionally place a heavy object when you are in need of extra strength or power.

Keep in mind that different types of stones or minerals are representative of different energies and intentions. What changes would you like to make in your life? What are you trying to achieve? Stones can assist in areas as diverse as romance, family, business, and luck. Do your research to identify which stones would be most suitable for your intentions.

Sound-Making Objects

Though using sound in Feng Shui seems like a temporary, short-lived action, sound can actually be a powerful tool that aids in clearing away harmful or stale energy, lifting the energy of a room, or calling in good luck. Bells, chimes, or singing bowls can provide clarity when you need it or increase mental alertness. Soothing background music can have a calming effect. As I mentioned in chapter 3, I keep a bell in the wealth area of my desk and ring it whenever I receive a check. I then place the check beneath the bell until it is ready to be deposited. This action improves the flow of money, but you can use bells to uplift or clarify any area of your life.

Bamboo flutes are also effective sound objects that are used in Feng Shui. Hanging flutes in your home can add strength and support, and they can increase your sense of security and peace. Placing bamboo flutes over a doorway provides protection to the area. Since bamboo is considered wood in Feng Shui, bamboo flutes take on the properties of the wood element. These elements include entrepreneurial energy, movement, and starting projects.

Water and Living Objects

Water objects are symbols of wealth and prosperity. Water can be free flowing and joyful, or it can be a powerful force of nature. Incorporating water objects into your home can be soothing and can create a suitable environment for reflection or meditation. Fountains or aquariums are examples of water features you could add to your space to promote abundance and rejuvenating energy.

Like water objects, living objects (such as houseplants and flowers) promote fresh, vibrant energy. Additionally, they symbolize growth and potential. Placing living objects in your space can also facilitate good luck. Just be sure your plants are positioned so they receive adequate sunlight—a dead plant (or even dried flowers) can stifle healthy chi.

Your Turn

Like a river, you are constantly changing as you pass through years and circumstances. Instead of fearing life's twists and turns, it is better to embrace them and look for opportunities amid the change. To get started, try the following activities:

1. **Engage in regular check-ins with yourself.**
   Using these check-ins, you can clarify your path and begin to understand how your surroundings are influencing you or holding you back from realizing your dreams.

2. **Use the following questions to guide you in self-reflection.**
   You can choose to silently answer the questions, speak your answers out loud, or jot down your thoughts in a notebook.

Ask yourself...

+ How have I been feeling lately? How would I *like* to be feeling?

+ What is my favorite area of my home or workplace? Why is it my favorite? What is the energy like in that room?

+ What are some areas of my house or workplace I avoid? Why do I avoid them? What is the energy like in those spaces?

+ Which areas could use decluttering or energy cleansing?

+ Does my home or office reflect who I am now? Does it reflect who I aspire to be? Or does it largely reflect the past?

+ Do I feel stifled or held back in any way? Why might that be?

+ What dreams or aspirations do I have for myself right now? Does my space need to be adjusted to better facilitate those dreams?

3. **Keep your self-reflection in mind when modifying your space.**

   If an area, object, or color no longer fits you, focus on changing it or letting it go. Use the insights you gained from the questions in step 2 to guide your adjustments.

Change does not have to be frightening. I challenge you to embrace it and look for the opportunities amid the transitions. When you dare to spread your wings and fly into new territory, you invite rejuvenating, vital energy into your life.

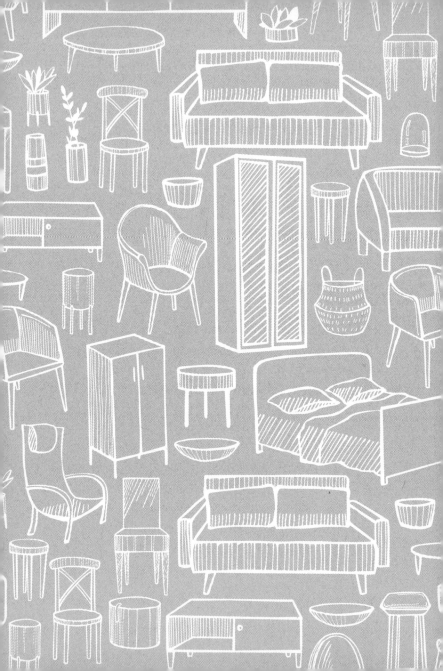

Chapter 11
Trusting the Process

Changing your space through Feng Shui and related practices is not the same as flipping a light switch. You may not experience profound changes or illumination right away—and even if you do, the space will likely need adjustments from time to time. Instead, modifying your space is more like building a bonfire. The kindling might not ignite right away, or it may need to be reconfigured. The larger pieces of firewood (i.e., major changes) need time and repeated exposure to the flame to catch. And once the bonfire is going, small adjustments and additions must be made to sustain the flame.

Just as patience, intentionality, and adjustments are required to build and sustain a fire, so, too, do these factors come into play in Feng Shui and other energy practices. There are times when an adjustment doesn't seem to "take" and one's aspirations are not immediately met. In these cases, it is a good idea to return to the basics and determine if a mistake was made in your intention. Sometimes, we tell ourselves falsehoods about what we want or hope to achieve (and sometimes we don't actually *know* what we want until we dive in and begin making changes). Additionally, if the occupant does not trust the process, that can affect the energy of the space and make goals or dreams much harder to achieve.

This chapter will discuss what to do if the changes made in a given space do not seem to be working. It will also touch upon some of the basic principles we've covered throughout this book and provide guidance on taking the next steps in your intentional design journey.

A Return to Basics

At its core, Feng Shui is not overly complicated. In addition to basic practices (clutter clearing, creating flow, etc.), it largely revolves around intentionality, trust, and visualizing your ideal future. Because we've covered a lot of ground in this book, I'd like to highlight some of the most important and essential ways to incorporate Feng Shui into your space. Even if you don't remember how to properly utilize a bamboo flute or position your dining room table, you can still achieve a successful design by paying attention to Feng Shui's foundational practices.

The following are my top five ways to use Feng Shui in your space:

1. **Clear the clutter.**

   A cluttered home or office can lead to myriad problems including stress, discomfort or unease, and the draining or stifling of energy. It can also cause you to remain stuck in the past and can inhibit forward movement.

Recently I visited a client in her home, where she had been living for decades. Before we began our work together, she had experienced a string of difficult and unsuccessful relationships, so I was not terribly surprised to discover that the relationship corner of her house (see the Bagua section for more) was filled to the gills with clutter. Items were piled on the table and crowding the floor. After I explained the negative effects this clutter could have, we set to work clearing the space and creating a welcoming corner for the energy to flow.

Keep in mind, shuffling the clutter off to the side or into a corner does *not* solve the problem. Instead, release the items that no longer serve you by donating, recycling, or discarding them. Create space for a new design and a new, more fruitful way of living.

2. **Create flow.**

In nature there is a natural flow. Vegetation and water work in tandem with the wildlife in a great give-and-take of resources. Wind streams through branches; water carves a path as it flows over rocks and minerals.

Similarly, it is possible to create a flow within the walls of your home or place of work. Pay attention to where people typically walk (the paths they take) and where they gather. Are there barriers blocking the natural flow? Do certain areas seem too crowded? When you intentionally open up your space, you invite natural, ever-present energy to flow through it.

3. **Balance the elements.**

It is essential to consider the five elements associated with Feng Shui practices when designing your space. These elements—fire, earth, metal, water, and wood—embody certain energies and are associated with particular colors, shapes, and images.

When the elements are in balance, they can positively affect the energy of a room—or even an entire home. When they are out of balance, they can create a sense of unease or anxiety. Additionally, the elements should reflect the occupants and nurture their dreams and desires.

The five elements can fall out of balance in a variety of ways. One common example is overrepresenting an element in a given space. Not long ago, I walked into a client's bathroom that was almost entirely white. Though the effect was clean and modern, it was also uncomfortable and felt harsh. Too much metal energy (represented by the color white) was present in the space, creating an off-kilter, unsettling feeling. To counter the over representation of an element, try incorporating other elements into the space. Wall paint, soothing artwork, a plant or two, or colorful accents are all ways to balance the space. I suggest introducing one or two new elements at a time (don't overdo it) to gently correct and adjust the area. If you need a refresher about the five elements and their properties, please refer to chapter 4.

4. **Utilize the Bagua.**
   The nine areas of the Feng Shui Bagua correspond to nine aspects of life: wealth, fame and reputation, marriage and partnerships, family, health, creativity and children, knowledge, career and life path, and helpful people and travel. We've already discussed how to use the Bagua grid to map out and adjust your space (see chapter 8), but I'd like to reiterate just how powerful and instrumental utilizing the Bagua can be. If a particular aspect of your life is suffering (or if you'd simply like to focus on improving a certain area), it is worth identifying that section on the Bagua chart and searching for ways to improve or amplify the energy in that space. It's a good idea

to focus on one or two areas at a time so your intentions *and* attention are not spread too thin.

Going back to my client with relationship problems, I identified the relationship corner of her home and immediately knew that area could be improved. In addition to excess clutter, there was also a cracked ceiling, a broken French door leading to an outdoor deck, old dishes, and unused furniture that she didn't care for. Many of the items in that area were hand-me-downs from other people or furnishings that had been purchased decades ago when she was still married to her husband. The predecessor energy that clung to these items felt heavy and was likely hindering her relationship success.

Fortunately, she was open to making changes (as I've mentioned before, intention is key), and we've been working together to adjust, rebalance, and improve her space.

5. **Reflect yourself and your dreams.**
   Above all, you should feel comfortable in your space. Let your unique self shine through as you select paint colors, choose artwork, or place accent pieces. Follow the Feng Shui guidelines, but don't be afraid to use your creativity and personal vision.

Some people are timid about artwork and have trouble choosing pieces for their space. That's a shame because artwork can truly be the soul of the room. It gives energy and life and can facilitate positive changes. When it comes to selecting artwork, I encourage using your intuition in tandem with Feng Shui best practices (such as balancing the five elements in a room).

Respected Feng Shui master and artist Carole Hyder talks about the parallels between Feng Shui and creating a painting. She encourages us to take remodeling projects (and paintings!) slowly. She says, "It's harder to get your intention and energy into something that's going full out. When you do it in phases, you have a chance to feel it out. Your intention can inform something—maybe there's another way to do it."[14]

As you're designing, remodeling, or adjusting your home or workplace, take it slow and regularly pause to consider how the space can serve your aspirations and goals. Who would you like to become in the coming year? What would you like to accomplish? Keeping these goals in mind, design a space that supports you *and* facilitates positive transformations.

---

14. Hyder, "Feng Shui & Art – A Conversation with Carole Hyder."

An Intentional Mindset

In addition to practicing Feng Shui basics to transform your space, it is critical to foster a mindset of intentionality and belief. If you harbor doubt or deem yourself unworthy of transformation, you're inviting negative energy to enter the space, and that can impede all progress. Instead, be open and accepting. Believe in possibilities!

My son Max embodies this spirit of openness and belief. Ever since he was a small child, he's had the natural ability to attract good things into his life. If he ever ran into a roadblock, he never fought it; instead, he pursued a different path. He always listened to his intuition.

Once, when I was sharing information about how to manifest desires, he stopped me and said, "Mom, don't you know? All you have to do is stay positive and believe." It's then I realized his soul already knew this truth, and he had been using these principles all along.

Sometimes, we can learn the simplicity of being open and believing in possibilities from our children. Embrace a child-like sense of wonder and peel back the layers of doubt and distrust. When you begin making adjustments in your home, make them intentionally and trust that the process will work if you follow basic Feng Shui principles and embrace a sincere, positive mindset.

Learn to listen to your intuition—that guiding energy that dwells within all of us. Your open, intentional, and intuitive spirit will be one of your greatest assets as you embark on your journey of changing your space and your life.

Signs and Symbols

When you open yourself to possibilities and welcome positive change, you create a space for signs and symbols to enter your life and guide you. Though many people do not realize it, these symbols come into our lives regularly, and it is up to us to slow down, open our hearts, and start seeing what we're meant to see.

When you live consciously and understand that energy is often manifested in symbols, you begin to see the world in a different way. You start to see the larger meaning in the little things that enter your life.

One winter, I was feeling particularly downtrodden because the weather was miserable and business was slower than usual, causing me to be short on money. Then, I had a dream in which I observed people smoking. I awoke excited, knowing that this was a powerful luck omen pertaining to prosperity. I took it as a sign that everything would be okay and money would soon come my way.

That same morning, I decided to take my time getting ready for work. I slowed down and thoroughly enjoyed the morning, even eating breakfast in my pajamas and taking time to read my horoscope. I left for work an hour and a half later than usual, and as I was in the car, I noticed a big eagle fly overhead. It swooped in close, and I could see its white head, big eyes, and yellow beak. It ended up following me for a quarter of a mile.

I knew this was no coincidence and that the eagle had entered my life for a reason. After a bit of research and talking to a few friends about the meaning of the eagle, I learned that eagles symbolize good luck, freedom, and the courage to look ahead—all messages I needed to hear.

Later that same day, I met with an artist in his gallery to view his artwork. We had been trying to meet for about nine months and had finally found time for our meeting. When I walked in, I was stunned to see a large framed photograph of a single eagle. I immediately understood that this synchronistic event was a sign and that I needed to take notice.

Upon returning home that day, I found an unexpected check from an insurance claim for one thousand dollars. It may have been unexpected, but it didn't surprise me one bit. I had witnessed signs throughout the day (and in my dreams) that gave me courage and implied that everything was going to be all right. And it was!

If you are open to receiving messages, they will come. However, you don't have to wait around, hoping a sign will cross your path. Facilitate what you need in your life through meditation, manifestation, and positivity. Remember the four-leaf clovers I mentioned in chapter 7? I beckoned these good-luck charms into my life by creating a space for them in my house—a little vase where they would be displayed. Another ritual I practice almost daily is lighting candles. You can purchase candles in any color and scent, and you can even burn candles that are specifically made to guide certain intentions (a romance candle, for instance, or a candle meant to bring in prosperity).

Signs, symbols, and omens can be powerful guides that can direct or comfort us. However, the most important factor is *you*. You must be open to receiving messages and trust your intuition when you think you've witnessed a sign or symbol. The same basic concept is true in your Feng Shui practice. Not every decision you make will be straightforward. At times, you simply have to pay attention to signs, trust your intuition, and move forward.

Trusting the Process

Trust and intuition come into play when you've made changes in your space and nothing seems to be happening. You might get frustrated and ask, "Why isn't this working? I thought changing my space was going to increase my prosperity," or "Why isn't my love life improving? I want results!"

In these cases, several factors could be contributing to a lack of progress or change. First of all, the answers you receive may not be obvious. It's possible someone new will come into your life who is *friends* with someone else who can help you. Or you might learn a new skill, which leads to discovering new people and possibilities. I experience chains of events like these on a regular basis.

Secondly, some changes take time. Even though certain transformations happen quickly (I've witnessed a few!), others need longer incubation periods. The change might happen incrementally and be so subtle you hardly notice it at first. It is important to trust the process and follow through to the end.

If, however, it becomes clear that changing your space has had little or no impact on your life, it's possible something else is amiss. Perhaps you're attempting to make too many changes at once and you need to gain greater focus around your goals and desires. Maybe your room or rooms are out of balance, and you need to rethink the layout, color schemes, or accessories. Or perhaps, minor adjustments need to be made with a mirror, heavy object, water feature, etc. to foster the kind of energy you'd like to create. Working with a Feng Shui interior designer can help you pinpoint any problematic areas and make the appropriate adjustments with good design in mind.

It's also possible to achieve precisely what you've intended … and then realize those intentions were not quite right. When we're manifesting something, we may *think* we know what is best for ourselves and our future, but once we achieve it, we may not be satisfied with the results. For example, that "dream job" you thought you wanted may end up being in a toxic work environment, or that "dream person" you wanted to attract may not actually be suited for you. To avoid this kind of disappointment, I advise broadening your intentions. Instead of fixating on a specific job, for instance, try meditating on prosperity and happiness in relation to your work. Instead of calling a specific person into your life, focus on beckoning a healthy relationship filled with love, respect, and joy. Broadening your intentions opens the door to many possibilities instead of just one. Try meditating on obtaining a certain feeling—peace, joy, contentment—instead of on a specific goal.

Your Turn

Ask yourself…

1. **What are some of the first steps I can take on my journey to transform my space?**
   Identify potential "problem areas" in your home or workspace that may be contributing to negative energy or stagnation. Is an area particularly cluttered? Do any of the objects, furnishings, or décor give you a sense of unease? How is the flow in the spaces where you live or work?

2. **How can I embrace an attitude of intentionality and openness?**
   Like a lotus flower, it is okay to open yourself slowly, petal by petal. Begin by accepting a few simple truths (e.g., "My intentions matter," "My

well-being is linked to my space," "Clutter and poor flow can negatively affect my attitude") and move on to embrace more complicated truths (e.g., the effectiveness of the Bagua, the way the five elements interact with each other). Keep an open mind as you begin your journey and don't worry if transformations do not happen overnight. Have faith that things will fall into place at the right time.

3. **Which feelings would I like to manifest for myself?**

   When you're modifying or adjusting a space, it is important to infuse it with your intentions. One way to do this is to focus on how you'd like to *feel* after the changes are made. Are you aiming for a more peaceful household? A workplace with acceptance and focus? A love life that is more harmonious and content? Visualize what life would be like if it were infused with these feelings.

Final Thoughts

F eng Shui is not magic. Instead, it is a recognition of our own truths and an expression of that truth within ourselves and our environment. Feng Shui and its related practices (such as biophilic design) help us to be happy with each other and comfortable in our own skins, to make our living spaces into homes that we love.

Feng Shui improves the flow of positive energy in a given space, which can have a profound impact on many areas of your life. The material world vibrates with energy—it is a part of every plant, every object, every rock or water fountain or coffee table. By changing certain design elements or placing certain objects into your space with intention, it is possible to shift the energy around you and begin to create a space that supports you and your aspirations.

At the core of Feng Shui is simplicity. When you live with simplicity, you can be more spontaneous, achieve a higher level of comfort, and find your inner calm. Simplicity—and its cousin, decluttering—involves scaling down and becoming mindful of each item you select for your space. Focus on purchasing a few high-quality items that fit with your room and your intentions rather than several lower-quality items chosen because they follow the latest trend.

As you go through life, remember you are an ever-changing being and it is vital for your living spaces to mirror who you are and who you aspire to become. When you sense it is time to let go, set aside time for mindful reflection and make a conscious effort to free up your energy and your space to make room for positive change.

When it comes to making changes (both in your space and within yourself), your intentions are of utmost importance. Be sincere and authentic on your Feng Shui journey. Any choices you make should follow Feng Shui principles, but they should also spring from your intuition and inner wisdom. You know and understand more than you realize.

Though intention is crucial, you must also be willing to commit and willing to take action. You do not have to tackle everything at once, but it's helpful to make a plan and start somewhere (again, listen to your intuition to determine where to center your focus). What actions are you willing to take *today* to make lasting changes tomorrow? You could choose to set aside time for quiet reflection or planning. Or you could commit to decluttering a certain area of your home. Or you might decide you need additional knowledge or support, which you could find by reading additional sources (see the recommended reading list in this book) or calling upon a Feng Shui interior designer, Feng Shui consultant, organizer, counselor, or healer.

You'll find that when you make intentional changes in your space, you will likely experience an array of emotional, relationship, and spiritual benefits. Here are a few results you may begin to notice:

+ Life tends to flow and it's easier to get "unstuck" if things go awry.
+ Dreams become reality.
+ Others tend to develop greater respect for you (reflecting the respect you've shown yourself) and your space.
+ You begin to feel calmer and more at peace.
+ You let things go, trusting in the forces that are greater than yourself.
+ Your gratitude grows.
+ You develop a deeper self-love.
+ You begin to love unconditionally.
+ Your compassion and empathy grow.
+ You become a more optimistic person.
+ Life begins to seem like a fun and interesting playground for you to enjoy.

I have witnessed profound changes take effect when people open their hearts and sincerely endeavor to make positive changes for themselves through intentionally modifying their spaces. Though Feng Shui is only one component of a complex, awe-inspiring universe, it is a powerful one. By applying its basic principles and making conscious choices, it is possible to tap into a wealth of energy and abundance. Your dreams *are* obtainable, and changing your space can help make them possible.

Recommended Reading

I n addition to looking over the following books, please consider visiting the website for my business, Metro Interiors, at MetroInteriors.com. There you will find a virtual portfolio along with a "Chapter Excerpts" section on the page dedicated to this book, which includes photos of some of the projects I've referenced. You will also find other valuable resources on the website, such as art and color tips, Feng Shui and Bagua basics, and a link to my newsletter.

Ask and It Is Given: Learning to Manifest Your Desires by Esther Hicks and Jerry Hicks

Breath: The New Science of a Lost Art by James Nestor

Buy Your Home Smarter with Feng Shui: Ancient Secrets to Analyze and Select Property Wisely by Holly Ziegler

Clear Your Clutter with Feng Shui: Free Yourself from Physical, Mental, Emotional, and Spiritual Clutter Forever by Karen Kingston

Complete Guide to Feng Shui Crystals by Terri Perrin

Conversations with Your Home: Guidance and Inspiration beyond Feng Shui by Carole J. Hyder

Creative Visualization: Use the Power of Your Imagination to Create What You Want in Your Life by Shakti Gawain

Diary of a Feng Shui Consultant and Visual Artist by Caroline Patrick BorNei

Fashion Feng Shui: The Power of Dressing with Intention by Evana Maggiore

Goal Achievement through Treasure Mapping: A Guide to Personal and Professional Fulfillment by Barbara J. Laporte

Infinite Possibilities: The Art of Living Your Dreams by Mike Dooley

The International Feng Shui Guild's Glossary of Universal Feng Shui Terms: A Guide for Practitioners and Enthusiasts by Lynne Ashdown, Rosalie Prinzivalli, and Yasha Jampolsky

Living Feng Shui: Personal Stories by Carole J. Hyder

Living in the Light: Follow Your Inner Guidance to Create a New Life and New World by Shakti Gawain

Love Is in the Earth: A Kaleidoscope of Crystals: The Reference Book Describing the Metaphysical Properties of the Mineral Kingdom by Melody

Make It Happen with Feng Shui: Attract What YOU Want! by Jen Leong

Meditations to Heal Your Life by Louise Hay

Move Your Stuff, Change Your Life: How to Use Feng Shui to Get Love, Money, Respect, and Happiness by Karen Rauch Carter

Personal Power through Awareness: A Guidebook for Sensitive People by Sanaya Roman

Playing the Matrix: A Program for Living Deliberately and Creating Consciously by Mike Dooley

Science of Breath: A Practical Guide by Swami Rama, Alan Hymes, and Rudolph M. Ballentine

Wind and Water: Your Personal Feng Shui Journey by Carole J. Hyder

You Can Heal Your Life by Louise Hay

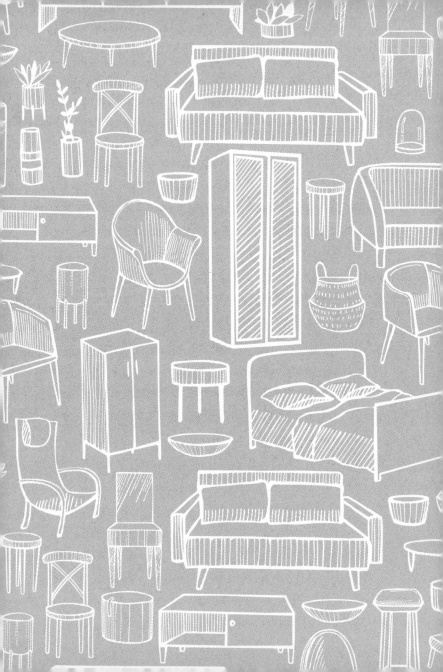

Bibliography

André, Christophe. "Proper Breathing Brings Better Health."
Scientific American. January 15, 2019. https://www
.scientificamerican.com/article/proper-breathing-brings
-better-health/.

Ashdown, Lynne, Rosalie Prinzivalli, and Yasha Jampolsky.
*The International Feng Shui Guild's Glossary of Universal
Feng Shui Terms.* Translated by Edgar Sung and Cindy
Chan. Lee's Summit, MO: International Feng Shui Guild,
2014.

"Bio for Oram Miller." Create Healthy Homes. Accessed November 14, 2022. https://createhealthyhomes.com/.

"Buildings & Built Infrastructure." Environmental and Energy
Study Institute. Accessed November 2, 2022. https://www
.eesi.org/topics/built-infrastructure/description#:~:text=
Any%20successful%20climate%20protection%20strategy
,of%20U.S.%20carbon%20dioxide%20emissions.

Goff, Sarah. "Asthma Facts and Figures." Asthma and Allergy
Foundation of America. Updated April 2022. https://
www.aafa.org/asthma-facts/.

Hyder, Carole. "Feng Shui & Art – A Conversation with Carole Hyder." By Julie Ann Segal. Metro Interiors. April 6, 2015. https://metrointeriors.com/2015/04/06/feng-shui-art-a-conversation-with-carole-hyder/.

Malik, Shiv. "Plants in Offices Increase Happiness and Productivity." *The Guardian*. https://www.theguardian.com/money/2014/aug/31/plants-offices-workers-productive-minimalist-employees. Accessed October 2021.

McGonigal, Kelly. "How to Create a Sankalpa." *Yoga International*. Accessed October 2021. https://yogainternational.com/article/view/how-to-create-a-sankalpa.

O'Toole, Garson. "Watch Your Thoughts, They Become Words; Watch Your Words, They Become Actions." Quote Investigator. January 10, 2013. https://quoteinvestigator.com/2013/01/10/watch-your-thoughts.

Rogers, Kara. "Biophilia Hypothesis." *Encyclopedia Britannica*. Updated June 25, 2019. https://www.britannica.com/science/biophilia-hypothesis.

Roman, Sanaya. *Personal Power through Awareness: A Guidebook for Sensitive People*. Novato, CA: New World Library, 2012.

Vallette, Jim, Rebecca Stamm, and Tom Lent. "Eliminating Toxics in Carpet: Lessons for the Future of Recycling." Healthy Building Network. October 26, 2017. https://healthybuilding.net/uploads/files/eliminating-toxics-in-carpet-lessons-for-the-future-of-recycling.pdf.

Wangdu, Lobsang, and Yolanda O'Bannon. "What Could Mean More? Om Mani Padme Hum." Yowangdu Experience Tibet. Updated August 5, 2020. https://www.yowangdu.com/tibetan-buddhism/om-mani-padme-hum.html.

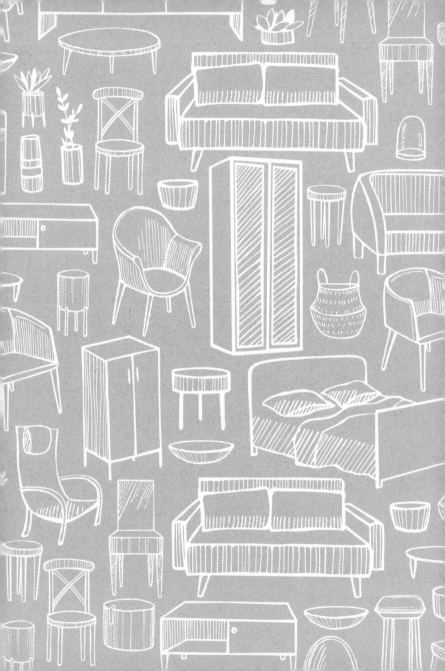

Notes

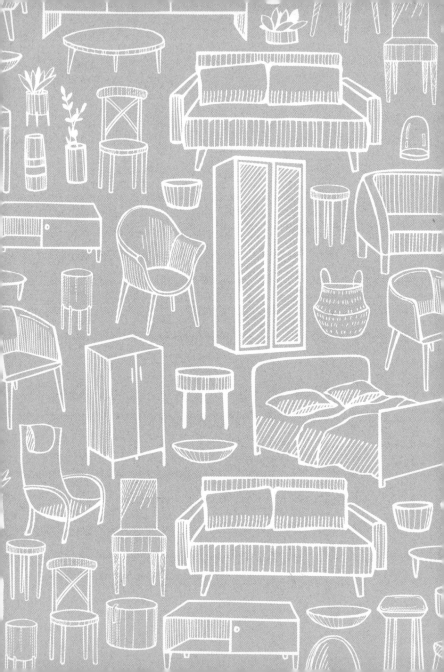

To Write to the Author

If you wish to contact the author or would like more information about this book, please write to the author in care of Llewellyn Worldwide Ltd. and we will forward your request. Both the author and the publisher appreciate hearing from you and learning of your enjoyment of this book and how it has helped you. Llewellyn Worldwide Ltd. cannot guarantee that every letter written to the author can be answered, but all will be forwarded. Please write to:

Julie Ann Segal
$^c/_o$ Llewellyn Worldwide
2143 Wooddale Drive
Woodbury, MN 55125-2989

Please enclose a self-addressed stamped envelope for reply,
or $1.00 to cover costs. If outside the U.S.A., enclose
an international postal reply coupon.

Many of Llewellyn's authors have websites with additional information and resources. For more information, please visit our website at http://www.llewellyn.com.

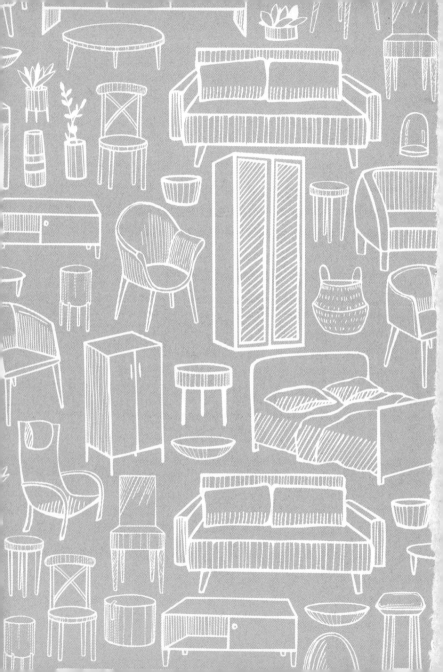